Essential Midwifery Practice:
Leadership, Expertise
and Collaborative Working

Dedication

This book is dedicated to all the midwives, students, colleagues, doctors, healthcare assistants, women and partners who have taught us all we know about leadership, collaboration and expertise.

Essential Midwifery Practice: Leadership, Expertise and Collaborative Working

Edited by

Soo Downe
RM, BSc, PhD

Sheena Byrom
RM, MA

Louise Simpson
RM, BA(Hons), MSc

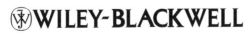

WILEY-BLACKWELL

A John Wiley & Sons, Ltd., Publication

This edition first published 2011
© 2011 Blackwell Publishing Ltd

Blackwell Publishing was acquired by John Wiley & Sons in February 2007. Blackwell's publishing programme has been merged with Wiley's global Scientific, Technical, and Medical business to form Wiley-Blackwell.

Registered office
John Wiley & Sons Ltd, The Atrium, Southern Gate, Chichester, West Sussex, PO19 8SQ, United Kingdom

Editorial offices
9600 Garsington Road, Oxford, OX4 2DQ, United Kingdom
2121 State Avenue, Ames, Iowa 50014-8300, USA

For details of our global editorial offices, for customer services and for information about how to apply for permission to reuse the copyright material in this book, please see our website at www.wiley.com/wiley-blackwell.

Wiley publishes its books in a variety of electronic formats: ePDF 9781444329230; ePub 9781444329247

Library of Congress Cataloging-in-Publication Data

Essential midwifery practice. Leadership, expertise and collaborative working/ edited by Soo Downe, Sheena Byrom, and Louise Simpson.
     p. ; cm.
  Other title: Expertise, leadership, and collaborative working
  Includes bibliographical references and index.
  ISBN 978-1-4051-8431-1 (pbk. : alk. paper)
  1. Midwifery. I. Downe, Soo. II. Byrom, Sheena. III. Simpson, Louise, RM.
IV. Title: Expertise, leadership, and collaborative working.
  [DNLM: 1. Midwifery. 2. Cooperative Behavior. 3. Leadership. 4.
Professional Competence. WQ 160 E779 2011]
  RG950.E64 2011
  618.2–dc22   2010022795

A catalogue record for this book is available from the British Library.

Set in 10/12.5pt, Palatino by Thomson Digital, Noida, India
Printed and bound in Singapore by Markono Print Media Pte Ltd.

1 2011

Contents

Contributors

Janet Baldwin is seconded to the NHS Institute of Innovation and Improvement UK as Clinical Lead on the Caesarean Section Team. In this role she works with midwifery and service improvement colleagues on a range of maternity improvements. She recently retired from clinical practice as a consultant obstetrician and gynaecologist at the West Middlesex University Hospital in London where she also held a succession of board-level posts, culminating in the Medical Directorship. In addition to Fellowships of the Royal College of Obstetricians and Gynaecologists and the Royal College of Physicians, she has a Master's degree in Healthcare Administration. She remains actively involved in clinical governance and undergraduate teaching for Imperial College London.

Alison Brodrick is a consultant midwife in normality at the Jessop Wing Sheffield Teaching Hospitals NHS Foundation Trust, UK. Prior to this she worked nationally as a midwife consultant to the Caesarean Section Team at the NHS Institute for Innovation and Improvement on projects in England and Wales, working with maternity service staff and users to optimise opportunities for normal birth. Having trained initially as a nurse, she qualified as a midwife in 1994 at Kingston upon Thames. Since then she has also worked as a lecturer practitioner with Nottingham University and as a midwife and supervisor of midwives with United Lincolnshire NHS Trust. Her strong focus on promoting normality and enabling change within maternity services was reflected in her Master's degree in Midwifery and in achieving an RCM award with a colleague in 2006.

Anna Byrom has worked within maternity services in the UK, as a midwife, for the past 6 years. She has worked around the UK within a range of midwifery care models, including a birth centre, working as a Sure Start caseload midwife and her present role as an infant feeding co-ordinator. Throughout her career, she has developed a philosophy of midwifery that embraces women's physical, emotional and social needs within the context of their family environment. She has a passion for social research and is currently undertaking a PhD with the University of Central Lancashire and the Maternal and Infant Nutrition and Nurture Unit. This research will involve exploring how macro-interventions impact on microcultures, looking specifically at UNICEF's Baby Friendly Hospital Initiative.

Sheena Byrom is Head of Midwifery at East Lancashire Hospitals Trust, UK. She qualified as a nurse and midwife in the 1970s, and has worked in the north of England since that time. Her past clinical practice encompasses 10 years within a GP unit, and then a combination of hospital and community midwifery, both clinical and managerial. Sheena worked as a consultant midwife for 6 years, in a role that encompassed the refocusing of maternity services in response to need, leading midwives in the public health agenda, and developing peer support networks and user involvement in service provision. Her post was part funded by the University of Central Lancashire where she contributed to the research capacity building strategy. Sheena was nominated twice to meet the Prime Minister, has been involved in several national projects with NICE and the Department of Health. She has published and presented nationally and internationally on topics such as addressing inequalities in health and promoting true woman-centred philosophies of care.

Ngai Fen Cheung is the professor and head of the first Chinese Midwifery Research Unit of the Nursing College of Hangzhou Normal University in China. Her main research interest is in the area of childbearing women's well-being and the development of Chinese midwifery. Her PhD, completed in the University of Edinburgh in 2000, compared the childbearing experiences of Chinese and Scottish women. Since then she has continued to design and organise international collaborative research projects studying Chinese midwifery. Her research aims to document and explain the practices of midwifery both in China and abroad, promoting normal birth and modern maternity care in China.

Sophie Cowley is an Associate with the NHS Institute for Innovation and Improvement, working on clinical pathway improvement. For the past 5 years she has supported NHS organisations delivering improvements in several pathways including promoting normal birth and reducing caesarean section rates, day surgery, radiology and ophthalmology. Previous to this Sophie was an information analyst with the NHS Modernisation Agency where she went on to become an improvement practitioner. Her main interests are service improvement tools and techniques, she has a Black Belt in Six Sigma and is currently studying for a Master's in Managing Quality in Health Care.

Ann Davenport A nurse since 1976 and midwife since 1991, Ann has been hired by organisations to live and work in more than 13 countries around the world – from the mountains of Nepal and Bolivia and the jungles of Brazil and Indonesia to the deserts of Ethiopia and western Mexico. She has worked with the University of Johns Hopkins Program for International Education in Gynecology and Obstetrics since 2001, along many other international organisations involved in the promotion of women and newborn health and well-being. She is the author of *Babies in the Cornfield: Stories of Maternal Life and Death from Around the World,* and lives in Chile, where she writes for a website promoting humanised childbirth (www.nuestroparto.cl).

Soo Downe leads the Research in Childbirth and Health (ReaCH) group at the University of Central Lancashire (UCLan) in England. Soo spent 15 years working as a midwife in various clinical, research and project development roles at Derby City General Hospital. In 2001 she joined UCLan, where she is now the Professor of Midwifery Studies. She currently chairs the UK Royal College of Midwives Campaign for Normal Birth steering committee, and she co-chairs the ICM Research Standing Committee. She has been a member of a number of national midwifery committees, and has held a number of visiting professorships, most recently in Belgium, Hong Kong, Sweden and Australia. Her main research focus is the nature of, and culture around, normal birth. She is the editor of *Normal Birth, Evidence and Debate* (2004, 2008), and the founder of the International Normal Birth Research conference series.

Kenny Finlayson has been working as a research assistant in the Research in Childbirth and Health (ReaCH) group at the University of Central Lancashire (UCLan) for the last 4 years. Although his background is in biochemistry and the pharmaceutical industry, Kenny has been involved in the research and practice of complementary medicine for much of the last decade. His research interests revolve around the integration of holistic approaches to healthcare, interprofessional boundary work and access to healthcare services by marginalised communities, all within a maternity context. For most of the last year Kenny has been deeply engaged in the design and development of a collaborative training programme for midwives and doctors. The programme is now entering its second phase of development and is being used as a regional initiative to foster a culture of collaboration within the maternity services.

Anita Fleming trained as a nurse and midwife in Blackburn, Lancashire, and has continued to work in East Lancashire since. After gaining all-round midwifery experience, Anita became a midwifery team leader in 2001. Having developed a particular interest in public health, she became a Sure Start midwife and in 2003 set up and led a midwifery group practice providing a caseload model of care to women from vulnerable groups. Anita is particularly interested in promoting normal birth and facilitating positive birth experiences for women, especially those deemed to be 'high risk', and this often involves working in collaboration with obstetricians to help enable this. She completed both a BSc(Hons) and MA in Midwifery at the University of Central Lancashire, and since February 2009, she has been working as a consultant midwife at East Lancashire Hospitals Trust and the University of Central Lancashire.

Sue Henry is Infant Feeding Co-ordinator at East Lancashire Hospitals NHS Trust, UK. Her current role focuses on leadership in the local maternity unit and primary care trust in reaching and maintaining full Baby Friendly Initiative standards, developing innovative ways to increase breastfeeding rates, and working closely with all partners and service users. Sue has represented her local trusts and shared her breastfeeding management experience via presentations and publications both regionally and nationally.

Lesley Kay is Lecturer in Midwifery at Anglia Ruskin University, UK. She previously worked as a midwifery team leader in a community-based team in the Cambridgeshire area. She completed a Master of Studies degree at the University of Cambridge in 2007, which incorporated the Postgraduate Certificate of Medical Education. She qualified as a midwife in 2000 after completing a direct-entry midwifery programme. In her current role, she is responsible for a 'Birth and Beyond' module, a 'Complexities' module and an 'Obstetric Challenges in Midwifery' module for the BSc(Hons) Pre-Registration Midwifery Pathway and the BSc(Hons) for Registered Nurses Pathway.

Nicky Mason is a midwife consultant seconded to the NHS Institute for Innovation and Improvement Caesarean Section Team in the UK. She has been a midwife since 1991 and has a background in clinical education and practice development. She has experience of facilitating large-scale change in both the south east of England and in Auckland, New Zealand through providing innovative coaching and support programmes to clinical staff. In her current role, Nicky has been working closely with maternity service staff and users across England and Wales to optimise opportunities for normal birth. Nicky is passionate about user involvement in service improvement and research. She has facilitated a women's focus group at her local unit since 2001 and is working with an advisory group of women who are supporting her in her PhD looking at women's narratives of planned caesarean birth.

Mary Newburn is Head of the NCT's Research and Information Team (RAIT). She is editor in chief of the NCT's continuing professional development journal, *New Digest*, and an advisor to the National Perinatal Research Unit. She trained as an NCT antenatal teacher before becoming a member of the NCT staff in 1988. Mary has a degree in sociology from the London School of Economics and a Master's degree in Public Health: Health Services Research from the London School of Hygiene and Tropical Medicine. She was made an honorary professor by Thames Valley University in 2004, awarded for services to midwifery and women's health.

Mary J. Renfrew is Professor and Director of the Mother and Infant Research Unit at York University. She is a graduate of the Department of Nursing Studies in the University of Edinburgh. She qualified as a midwife in 1978 and gained her PhD in Edinburgh in 1982 while working with the Medical Research Council Reproductive Biology Unit. She has since worked in Oxford, Alberta, Canada, Leeds and York. She established and led the Midwifery Research Initiative at the National Perinatal Epidemiology Unit, and has been co-editor of the Cochrane Pregnancy and Childbirth Group. She established the multidisciplinary Mother and Infant Research Unit (MIRU) in 1996. Her research has been funded by the Medical Research Council, the Department of Health, the National Institute for Health Research, the National Institute for Health and Clinical Excellence and the ESRC, among others. In addition to more than 90 academic journal publications, she has written widely about maternity care, and is author or editor of seven books, including *A Guide to Effective Care in Pregnancy and Childbirth* with Murray Enkin, Marc Keirse and Jim Neilson. She has an active interest in the integration of research, education, policy and practice, and has worked closely with service users and consumer groups for many years. She has sat on committees at national and international level including Chair of the WHO Strategic Committee for Maternal and Newborn Health. She has been awarded inaugural Senior Investigator status by the National Institute for Health Research.

Louise Simpson is Practice Education Facilitator, Women's, Children and Sexual Health Division, Mid Cheshire NHS Trust, Crewe. She has been a practising midwife for 10 years. She has also worked as a labour ward co-ordinator. Her current role is to promote leaning within the clinical environment, and to support midwives in a clinical capacity. Her philosophy of care is to promote pregnancy, labour and birth as a normal, natural process placing emphasis on birth as a whole, and supported through attending to the physical, social and emotional needs of the woman and her family. Louise is passionate about midwifery and research. She was involved in the data collection for the RCM

'Campaign for Normal Birth'. Her Master's by research explored midwives' accounts of intrapartum expertise. Through this research, she identified the skills, practices and personal attributes required to promote expertise in practice. She has presented the findings of this research at local, national and international conferences, and published her findings in leading journals.

Denis Walsh is Associate Professor in Midwifery, University of Nottingham, UK. He was born and brought up in Queensland but trained as a midwife in Leicester, UK, and has worked in a variety of midwifery environments over the past 25 years. His PhD was on the birth centre model. He lectures on evidence and skills for normal birth internationally and is widely published on midwifery issues and normal birth. He authored the best seller *Evidence-Based Care for Normal Labour and Birth*.

Cathy Warwick CBE is General Secretary of the Royal College of Midwives (RCM), one of the world's oldest and largest midwifery organisations, representing the majority of the UK's midwives. She has written and published widely on midwifery issues and lectures and speaks nationally and internationally. She was awarded a visiting professorship by King's College, London in 2004. She received a CBE for services to healthcare in 2006, and was awarded an Honorary Doctorate from St George's and Kingston University, London, in 2007.

Foreword

This book addresses three aspects of midwives' work: leadership, expertise and collaboration. Individually, each is important to describing midwifery practice; collectively, they are a dynamic package that can elevate the health of women and babies locally and across the broad global community.

Midwives are called upon to be many things to many people. They must be first-rate practitioners who use their knowledge, skill and expertise to care effectively for women and babies. Some would say that is enough and all that really counts. But it is not! Students and junior midwives often funnel their energy into developing skills, as they should. However, their vision should not be so narrow as to block out other important aspects of midwifery practice. They must realise that their practice reflects the environment in which they work and the world in which we all live. They have the potential to influence both for the good of mothers and babies. This requires commitment to developing expert clinical skills, but also to broadening their expertise as collaborators and leaders.

As we all know, there are many paths, venues, roadblocks and bridges in the birth journey. Navigating that 'travail' (journey/the work of labour) is something a woman does in concert with others and she deserves the very best artists who are in harmony *with her* in the process. Her midwife should be a practitioner who artfully collaborates with others to ensure that the woman's needs are met. Skilled collaboration fosters seamless care transitions when required, integrates complex healthcare systems and opens closed doors. Collaboration among practitioners involved in childbearing care is essential, but collaboration with the woman and family and the broad community also is important. It is a skill and not always easy, especially within daunting hierarchal institutions. It requires the recognition that all who enter a collaborative relationship are human beings with individual beliefs and values shaped by their culture, education and experiences. If we pride ourselves (as we often contest) that we are listeners and value each woman as an individual then it is incumbent upon all of us to apply those same communication skills and beliefs to the development of our collaborative professional and community relationships.

Leadership is perhaps the part of the job description that is shunned by many midwives who think, 'I just take care of women – I don't need to be a leader!'. But you are and you do – you just may not realise the form it takes or the far-reaching impact it can have. Leadership goes further than the common misperception of a leader as the lofty head of a group, institution or country. Rather, it is the everyday work that demonstrates strength, knowledge and ethical behaviour to others. Your actions should be those that others want to emulate. This means being engaged in work to further the health of mothers and babies, as an individual and as a member of the broader community – you are part of the solution!

This book will help you learn about and reflect on these vital aspects of our work and how you can develop each of them as a midwife. As I reflect on my own midwifery path, I have come to realise that all of these have added to the joy and challenges of my work. Although the path was never easy, the forward journey and navigating the pitfalls have added to the richness of my professional life. If we all embrace these aspects of our work, the world will become a better place for mothers, babies, families and the broader global community.

Holly Powell Kennedy PhD, CNM, FACNM, FAAN
Helen Varney Professor of Midwifery
Yale University School of Nursing
New Haven, Connecticut, USA
holly.kennedy@yale.edu

Introduction

Soo Downe, Sheena Byrom and Louise Simpson

Leadership, expertise and collaborative working are fundamental aspects of efficient and effective healthcare. These three aspects have been recognised in governmental and health agency documents across the world (WHO 2005; DH 2007a). While there has been some exploration of these areas in the nursing literature, there is a paucity of theoretical and practical exploration of the nature and application of these characteristics in the context of maternity care. This book offers a comprehensive overview of the general theories, principles and points of good practice in each of these three areas. This general literature is then contextualised by theoretical and practical implications for maternity care. Each section is illustrated with in-depth case studies of successful innovation and change in practice based on the theories and concepts discussed in earlier chapters.

Leadership

The World Health Organization (WHO) recognises the importance of strong leadership for effective healthcare. The WHO has also developed a programme for potential dynamic leaders in an attempt to combat poverty and health inequalities (WHO 2005). In the UK, the Department of Health has developed a leadership centre as part of the NHS Modernisation Agency, in the belief that leaders within the NHS could motivate staff and improve patient care (DH 2003).

Essential Midwifery Practice: Leadership, Expertise and Collaborative Working, first edition. Edited by Soo Downe, Sheena Byrom and Louise Simpson
Published 2011 by Blackwell Publishing Ltd.
© 2011 Blackwell Publishing Ltd.

Examination of the literature on leadership and that relating to midwifery reveals some evolutionary similarities. The dominant theories in both areas appear to be moving away from hierarchical models and towards those based on relationship. In the case of leadership, this has led to a concentration on transformational philosophies, in contrast to earlier approaches based on command and control (Conger 1991; Barker 1994; Carless 1998). In midwifery, woman-centred care has become the ideology of choice, theoretically replacing hierarchies built on professional power bases (WHO 1997; DfES 2004; DH 2007b). The leadership section of the book examines the theoretical synergies between these two movements and provides examples of effective leadership in practice.

Expertise

It is not uncommon for midwives to call themselves 'the experts in normal childbirth'. The statement appears to see both 'expertise' and 'normality' as unproblematic concepts. In many countries across the world, the majority of women giving birth with trained midwives currently do not experience a physiological birth. This raises questions about the nature and provenance of expert or exemplary practice in midwifery. The section on expertise will draw on general theories of expertise, on established usage of the term in nursing and medicine, on emerging theories in midwifery, and on practical examples of expertise in practice through in-depth case studies Given the fact that most women in the world are not attended by trained midwives, this section also addresses the topic of maternity care expertise for practitioners without formal midwifery qualifications.

Collaborative working

The concept of increased inter- and/or multidisciplinary collaboration is advocated by various governing bodies. In a recent document entitled *Safer Childbirth: Minimum Standards for Service Provision and Care in Labour* (RCOG, RCM, RCA, RCPCH 2007), a range of UK professional bodies comment that national audits and reviews of maternity services have continued to highlight poor outcomes related to multiprofessional working, staffing and training (Foreword). The NHS Institute for Innovation and Improvement has defined four levels of collaboration (DH 2007b). This section will explore the roots of effective and ineffective collaborative working, summarise the key theories, concepts and policy documents in this area, and present case studies from the UK and China to illustrate how collaboration across professional and agency boundaries can be improved, and the implications this has for practice and for outcomes.

Conclusion

Strategic and clinical leadership, the application of expertise and effective intra- and interprofessional collaboration are essential components in the provision of high-quality healthcare. We hope that this book will assist midwives, midwifery students at all levels, and others working in or studying maternity care to understand the theoretical underpinnings of effective leadership, expertise and collaborative ways of working. We also aim to inspire positive changes in practice, through the provision of inspirational case studies of change and innovation. We hope this text is a practical guide to such change for the future.

References

Barker AM (1994) An emerging leadership paradigm: transformational leadership. In Hein EC, Nicholson MJ (eds) *Contemporary Leadership Behavior: Selected Readings*, 4th edn. Philadelphia, J B Lippincott.

Carless SA (1998) Gender differences in transformational leadership: an examination of superior, leader, and subordinate perspectives. *Sex Roles: A Journal of Research* 39(11-12). www.findarticles.com (accessed June, 2010).

Conger JA (1991) Inspiring others: the language of leadership. *Academy of Management Executive* 5(1).

Department for Education and Skills (2004) *National Service Framework for Children, Young People and Maternity Services*. London, Department for Education and Skills. www.dh.gov.uk/en/Publicationsandstatistics/ Publications/PublicationsPolicyAndGuidance/DH_4089114 (accessed June, 2010).

Department of Health (2003) The Leadership Centre. http://webarchive .nationalarchives.gov.uk/+/www.dh.gov.uk/en/Managingyourorganisation/ Humanresourcesandtraining/Modelcareer/DH_4080689 (accessed June, 2010).

Department of Health (2007a) *Maternity Matters: Choice, Access and Continuity of Care in a Safe Service*. London, Department of Health.

Department of Health (2007b) Institute for Innovation and Improvement. *Delivering Quality and Value: Focus on Caesarean*. www.institute.nhs.uk/ quality_and_value/introduction/toolkits_for_high_volume_care_pathways .html (accessed June, 2010).

Department of Health (2007c) Institute for Innovation and Improvement. www .nhsleadershipqualities.nhs.uk/ (accessed June, 2010).

RCOG, RCM, RCA, RCPCH (2007) *Safer Childbirth: Minimum Standards for Service Provision and Care in Labour*. www.rcog.org.uk/files/rcog-corp/uploaded-files/WPRSaferChildbirthReport2007.pdf (accessed June, 2010).

World Health Organization, Department of Reproductive Health and Research (1997) *Care in Normal Birth: A Practical Guide.* Geneva, World Health Organization.

World Health Organization (2005) The Health Leadership Service. www.who .int/health_leadership/en/ (accessed June, 2010).

Part I
Leadership

Introduction to Part I

Sheena Byrom

The subject of leadership in general has received much attention throughout the world. Although there is a significant amount of research and expert opinion in relation to leadership and health professionals, there has been less examination of the issues relating to leadership and the midwifery profession.

Examination of the literature on leadership and that relating to midwifery reveals some evolutionary similarities. The dominant theories in both areas appear to be moving away from hierarchical models and towards those based on relationship. The emotional focus of midwifery work, and the philosophy of women-centred care where midwives support and nurture women, could be linked with transformational style leadership theory. While it has been suggested that there is a lack of effective midwifery leadership across the world, there are examples of midwifery leaders who are challenging that belief, through their dynamic leadership styles, in strategic development, midwifery research, education, academia and service provision.

In Chapter 1, Sheena Byrom and Lesley Kay examine the general and specific literature relating to leadership theory. They provide a brief overview of various leadership styles and traits. The subject of whether leaders are born or made is debated, in addition to various approaches to leadership development. There is an agreement within the literature that leadership is an essential element of organisational success, and for maternity services leadership has been identified as a critical factor when considering optimum safety for mothers and babies. The chapter suggests that all midwives have a responsibility to 'lead' in certain circumstances – for example, they 'lead' women during the childbirth continuum in their daily work, they lead parent education sessions, and they facilitate birth. The chapter proposes that the way midwives 'lead' women or other midwives needs to be considered at all times if quality of care is to be improved.

Sheena Byrom, Soo Downe and Anna Byrom take a more theoretical approach in Chapter 2, in which they describe a 'nested narrative review' of the literature pertaining to midwifery, woman-centred care and transformational leadership theory. Midwives and midwifery have always championed a holistic approach to childbirth. Even though transformational leadership has been closely linked to feminine traits by some authors, there appears to be little in the literature about the possibility of adopting transformational leadership approaches in midwifery. The chapter reviews the literature of woman-centred care and transformational leadership separately. On the back of the findings, it is suggested that the two approaches have much in common. The authors suggest that adoption of transformational leadership styles may be welcomed, at least in some midwifery settings.

A series of case studies and personal reflections are set out in Chapter 3. Contributions include personal reflections from midwifery leaders working at various levels. Sue Henry, Sheena Byrom and Cathy Warwick offer insights from the UK as midwives working at local level, as a consultant midwife and as a national leader, respectively. Ngai Fen Cheung gives an example of leading radical change in China, and a service user leader, Mary Newburn, describes how she came to a position of national influence in maternity care. Individuals frequently describe being inspired by leaders. The chapter provides personal insights into how such people achieve their vision and their ultimate success. Their skill and capacity to develop others to succeed and their influence on maternity service development offer encouragement and inspiration to all midwives, now and in the future.

Chapter 4, written by Mary Renfrew, uses the subject of breastfeeding as a case study to examine ways of creating change at a wide range of levels, from the very local to the international. Mary describes ways in which her work has attempted to address challenges faced in terms of research, practice, policy, education and strategy. Crucially, she draws out lessons for leadership in creating change at scale. The chapter highlights the fact that success depends on all members of the team, each bringing their contribution, skills, expertise and talents. Mary is clear that successful leadership includes having the confidence to ask others to follow, and the ability to work in collaboration and to follow others in turn.

All the chapters in this section illustrate the need for courage, vision and conviction if leaders are to be effective. They set out the theoretical basis for leadership and provide examples of where good leadership has led to important changes at all levels. As such, they provide a set of principles and a series of templates for midwifery leaders in the future.

Chapter 1
Midwifery Leadership: Theory, Practice and Potential

Sheena Byrom and Lesley Kay

Introduction

In 2008 the World Health Organization (WHO 2008) highlighted consistent leadership as a vital element to improve maternal, newborn and child health, and as a crucial component for progress towards Millennium Development Goals 4 and 5. Whilst this is a global strategy, many countries are also individually promoting positive leadership as key to promoting safe and appropriate maternity care.

This chapter will provide an overview of theory underpinning the concept of leadership, with a particular focus on maternity services and midwifery care. It provides the reader with a basic insight into the current position of leadership within maternity services, and into the potential for improvement and implications for the future. Whilst reference is made to other countries the majority of the examples of current practice apply to the UK.

Leadership and leaders: theory, styles and traits

Leadership theory has been debated for centuries throughout the world, and yet it remains difficult to give a precise and agreed definition to the word 'leadership' (Mullins 2009). Put simply, it could be described as a relationship through which one person influences the behaviour or actions of other people in the accomplishment of a common task (Mullins 2009).

Essential Midwifery Practice: Leadership, Expertise and Collaborative Working,
first edition. Edited by Soo Downe, Sheena Byrom and Louise Simpson
Published 2011 by Blackwell Publishing Ltd.
© 2011 Blackwell Publishing Ltd.

The concept of leadership is related to motivation, communication and interpersonal skills (Tack 1984) and has been suggested as the critical variable in defining the success or failure of an organisation (Schein 2004). Successful leaders have emerged within community groups, religious circles, political arenas and armed forces, and their talents have ranged from leading a few individuals to leading whole countries.

It could be useful to consider the following suggestions from Anderson *et al.* (2009) when trying to navigate the leadership phenomenon.

- Leadership (and management) is about dealing with the boundary between order and chaos – management leans more towards the order side and leadership more towards the chaos/complexity side. The issue is to balance the maintenance of what is useful (unless it is dysfunctional) while developing the new, and managing the transitions from one state to another.
- Leadership has become much more prevalent as a word and concept and has taken over from management, important in the era of manufacturing.
- Good management is added to, not replaced, by leadership. Well-led change needs good management to implement and maintain it.
- Leadership as an activity has in recent years been seen to be more distributed. Although it is still seen as the responsibility of a significant few, it is also a concern of the many who can have significant impact. Leadership is in part about human capital, contained in individuals, but also partly about social capital, embedded in collectives and their relationships: teams, networks, whole organisations and even sectors and regions. This presents real challenges for leadership development.

Leadership is an integral part of the social structure and culture of an organisation (Mullins 2009). When contemplating organisational culture, consideration should be given to how leaders create culture, and how culture defines and creates leaders (Schein 2004). Interestingly, and relevant to this chapter, the Care Quality Commission (2008), in its survey of all UK maternity services, reported that poor morale and ineffective or authoritarian leadership are commonly linked. The Commission noted that this is likely to contribute to a less effective service. It recommended that hospital organisations (trusts) need to consider the culture within their maternity services.

The so-called 'Great Man' and 'Trait' theories were the basis for most leadership research until the mid-1940s (Bednash 2003) These theories suggest that leaders are born and not made, and that leaders possess certain innate qualities or characteristics such as interpersonal skills, judgement and fluency (Bass 1990). Contemporary opponents of these theories (Cook 2001; Gould *et al*. 2001) argue that leadership skills can be developed and are not necessarily inborn. Handy (1993) describes a major flaw of the trait theories: they disregard the influence of others or the situation on the leadership role. Trent (2003) agrees, maintaining that leadership requires collaborators more than charisma.

Vroom & Yetton (1973) and later Vroom & Jago (1988) developed a model called situational contingency theory. This theory considers how and the degree to which the leader engages his or her team members in the decision-making process (Vroom & Jago 2007). It suggests that the same leader can use different group decision-making approaches depending on the characteristics of each situation. 'Style' theory succeeded both trait and situational theories and concentrates on what effective leaders actually do as opposed to what sort of person they are. Leadership in this context is understood as a set of behaviours rather than a set of traits.

Lewin *et al*. (1990) undertook seminal work on leadership styles. They considered some leaders' need to demonstrate a degree of dictatorial authority as opposed to the readiness of other leaders to assume a more democratic role. Leaders taking an autocratic stance make decisions without consulting others. Ralston (2005) describes this type of style as 'authoritarian'. Communication is top-down and staff are not expected or encouraged to take the initiative. In contrast, in the democratic style, the leader involves others in decision making and is often described as 'participative'. This is usually appreciated by people and improves staff morale and ownership; however, problems can arise when there is a wide range of opinions and there is no clear way of reaching an equitable decision. In another approach, the *laissez-faire* style of leadership minimises the leader's involvement in decision making. Those of this ilk tend to lead by virtue of their position in the organisation, without necessarily displaying leadership skills (Ralston 2005).

Burns (1978) conceptualised leadership in terms of a leadership–member exchange model, a two-directional process between follower and leader. This differentiates between transactional and transformational leadership styles. Transactional leadership occurs when one person takes the initiative in making contact with others for the purpose of making an exchange (Conger & Kanungo 1994), whereas transformational leaders communicate positive self-esteem and empowerment of followers (Davidhizar 1993).

Transformational leadership

The leadership style that is increasingly advocated in the healthcare literature is that based on the transformational model (Kouzes & Posner 2007). Ralston (2005, p.35) defines transformational leadership as 'inspirational and empowering, challenging thinking and offering informal rewards at every opportunity'. Coggins (2005) suggests that leaders using this model tend to motivate others to apply their own leadership behaviours. The transformational leader attempts 'to engage the full person as the follower' (Ralston 2005, p.35).

Some have argued that transformational leadership styles have parallels with feminist theories, specifically where they act to empower women (Helgesen 1990; Coggins 2005). Indeed, Helgesen describes a set of feminine principles which are argued to guide women's typical leadership behaviour: caring, being involved, helping, being responsible, making intuitive decisions and structuring organisations as networks rather than hierarchies.

Transformational leadership is well established in the literature. One of the most clearly articulated and rigorously tested contributions is the 'five practices of exemplary leadership' model (Table 1.1) (Kouzes & Posner 2007). In 1983, Kouzes and Posner set out to establish what it was that leaders did when they realised their personal best in leading rather than managing others (Van Maurik 2001). The five key elements Kouzes and Posner describe are elemental practices that enable leaders to get things done. According to Kouzes and Posner, leadership starts where

Table 1.1   The five key elements of transformational leadership (Kouzes & Posner 2007). Descriptors added by Kay (2007)

Element	Descriptor
Challenging the process	• Break new ground • Search for the potential to progress and evolve • Prepared to take the risk of failing
Modelling the way	• Act as a role model • Be transparent about vision and values • Act consistently within those values
Inspiring a shared vision	• Exhibit belief and enthusiasm • Enlist and motivate others
Encouraging the heart	• Acknowledge contributions • Celebrate achievements
Enabling others to act	• Establish trust • Build strong relationships • Engage everyone involved • Empower others

management ends and where 'systems of control, reward, incentive and overseeing give way to innovation, and where individual character and courage of convictions can achieve great things' (Van Maurik 2001, p.109). Leadership, they argue, is not about personality but about behaviour and relationships.

Leadership characteristics and traits

Pashley (1998) suggests that, on the basis of research, theory and practice, the range of prescriptive characteristics, qualities and skills that can be attributed to a leader is vast. Kouzes and Posner's (2007) research, for example, single-handedly recognised 255 characteristics of leadership. In their study profiling nursing leaders, Antrobus and Kitson (1999, p.750) identified common themes from the interview data which enabled them to outline the 'skills repertoire' of the 'future nurse leader' (Box 1.1).

Box 1.1   Leadership traits identified by Antrobus and Kitson (1999)

- A powerful influential operator – empowering relationships created with others

- A strategic thinker – creating meaning and supporting learning

- A developer of nursing knowledge – assimilating research evidence with practice

- A reflexive thinker – having a clear understanding of values, purpose and personal meaning

- A process consultant – working through and with others to achieve transformational change

---

Although it is not clearly stated in the research report, the inference is made that leadership relates to occupying a certain hierarchical status within an organisation. On the other hand, Christian and Norman (1998) identified ten elements that are central to the clinical leader role at all levels. This core set of attributes was considered applicable across clinical settings and specialties. In addition to co-ordinating and managing abilities, the core characteristics included encouraging staff ownership of changed practices as well as enabling staff development, supporting and motivating the team, networking, and acting as a change agent. In their report, the authors summarize the data by outlining a 'profile' of a nurse development unit clinical leader. Although this makes for an interesting read, there is no clear explanation in the text of how this profile was determined; it is therefore difficult to see how the core set of attributes can be applicable across settings and specialties.

An understanding of the constraints on clinical leaders, especially in relation to their position in the organisational hierarchy, emerged from Christian and Norman's (1998) study. Those without managerial responsibility who had the potential to produce a vision for the future lacked authority to make it happen, and those who had managerial authority at a strategic level could not extricate themselves from administration to be creative in clinical practice.

Conversely, Stanley's study of clinical leaders in paediatric nursing (2004, p.42) determined that clinical leadership, in this specific setting, was not tied to a hierarchical position and that clinical leaders are seen as nursing staff who are 'able to be supportive, cope well with change in the clinical environment ... guide, motivate, act as an advocate, inspire confidence, think critically and remain clinically competent'. According to Stanley (2004), the study demonstrates that clinical nurse leaders exist across the gamut of nursing grades, principally in relation to nurses with a strong clinical focus. Stanley does acknowledge, however, that the study findings could be limited by the fact that the participants were settling in to new surroundings (which could have affected their responses).

Leadership and health services: the UK example

Both leadership and quality improvement are high on the National Health Service (NHS) agenda in the UK. Appropriate and effective leadership is critical to the transformation and improvement of health care (Reinertsen *et al.* 2008; Health Foundation 2009a,b), with consideration given to both clinical and strategic leadership. For health-care organisations in particular, leadership capabilities need to be nurtured and expanded at all levels, and within all professions. Indeed, David Nicholson, Chief Executive Officer for the NHS (NHS 2009), proclaimed:

> We are extremely lucky to already have fantastic leaders throughout the National Health Service. But if we are to realise our vision of an NHS that puts quality at the heart of everything it does, we need to embrace more leaders from all levels in the service and from a wider range of backgrounds.

For midwives, other professionals and citizens of the UK, there are programmes of learning for aspiring leaders, and established pathways to recognise those who demonstrate exceptional capabilities (Cabinet

Office 2009; NHS 2009). In 2009, the UK's Department of Health established a National Leadership Council (DH 2009a) to assist with implementing actions from the final report of Lord Darzi's Next Stage Review (DH 2009b). This document is clear in its support for, and championing of, leadership in the NHS and has a clear framework for delivering the agenda (Dawson *et al.* 2009). Part of the remit for the Council is to seek transformational change in the culture of leadership, with much emphasis on encouragement, support and mentoring.

Maternity care and midwifery leadership

It has been suggested that there is a lack of midwifery leadership in other countries too, and the International Confederation of Midwives (ICM) has set up a Young Midwifery Leadership Programme to address this (ICM 2010). Specifically, the UK Department of Health has suggested that the lack of midwifery positions at a senior level within some UK hospitals may have contributed to poor quality of care (DH 2009b).

> The ability of midwives to be strategic leaders in service, policy and higher education requires that these roles are there to start with; and that midwives have the expertise, credibility and leadership skills to represent our profession and its contributions.
>
> (DH 2009c, p.32)

This statement is taken directly from a recent UK midwifery directive, and captures in one paragraph the current situation in relation to UK midwifery leadership. The document describes the importance of the midwifery contribution to the maternity governance agenda, and suggests that when there is midwifery influence at board level, it enhances the opportunity for midwifery leaders to engage in decisions about strategies and systems that meet the needs of women and their families. Within the UK, midwifery leaders are evident to some degree in strategic, academic and direct service positions. Professors of midwifery, consultant midwives, heads of midwifery and the General Secretary position at the Royal College of Midwives are strategic roles, and many of the individuals in those roles have influence at a national and international level. In addition, midwives lead teams, including those that are multidisciplinary, and there are others demonstrating leadership capabilities through their clinical work as midwives. Even so, there is a perceived lack of leadership in maternity services in the UK, and this has been highlighted in reports relating to the safety agenda (Care Quality Commission 2006; King's Fund 2008).

As with general healthcare, leadership within maternity services needs to occur at all levels and within each element of the multidisciplinary team. For maternity services, the evidence in relation to the

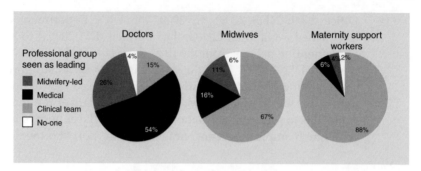

Figure 1.1 Perceptions of sources of leadership in the maternity unit by professional group. Source: HCC (2008) survey of Maternity staff 2007.

safety of maternity services highlights difficulties with leadership and management, stating that maternity teams are not always clear about leadership and are not always well managed (King's Fund 2008). In addition, in 2006 a report on the investigation into ten maternal deaths in one UK maternity service revealed a distinct lack of leadership (Care Quality Commission 2006).

As midwifery-led care expands within the UK, there is increasing debate as to who 'leads' the management of maternity care overall. The Care Quality Commission (2008) asked members of maternity teams throughout the UK who led maternity care. Rather worryingly, both midwives and medical staff perceived that it was their professional group (Figure 1.1). This result could be viewed as lack of defined leadership or a deficit in understanding of roles in general. It could also be the result of lack of team work, collaboration and shared goals, and suggests a continuation of the historical pursuit of power and control between professional groups and hierarchies (Donnison 1988).

The recent King's Fund *Safe Births* document (King's Fund 2008) maintains that healthcare is in the process of moving away from a traditional hierarchical model of organisation and leadership towards a team approach, which should include midwifery supervisors, managers, consultant midwives, educationalists and other professionals. A strong, integrated team enhances the capacity of clinical midwives to offer flexible and relevant woman-centred care. In her seminal book on effective teamwork, West (2004) suggests that traditional leaders tend to direct rather than facilitate and support, to give rather than seek advice and to determine rather than integrate views. Current UK policy on maternity services reminds maternity care workers of the excellent opportunities to work in partnership with the leads of other professional groups, such as non-clinical managers and midwives, and in leadership positions in other sectors, such as policy bodies and universities (DH 2009a). Ralston (2005) is of the opinion that this is happening in practice, and that the delivery of midwifery care is changing from a task-oriented approach to a team approach, where midwives collaborate with others to provide holistic care. Chapter 9 debates the benefits of collaborative working in maternity services in more detail.

The Care Quality Commission's (CQC) monitoring of maternity services (Care Quality Commission 2008) highlights considerable variations in quality of care received by women across the UK. Pressure groups such as the Association for Improvements in Maternity Services (AIMS: see www.aims.org.uk) and the National Childbirth Trust (see www.nctpregnancyandbabycare.com/home) are continually striving to improve quality within maternity care systems. It is imperative that all midwives understand their leadership role in the delivery of high-quality care, on a day-to-day basis. It could be argued that midwives 'lead' women during the childbirth continuum in their daily work, leading parent education sessions, for example, and facilitating birth. The way midwives 'lead' women or other midwives needs to be considered at all times if quality of care is to be improved. Byrom and Downe's (2010) research suggests that to become effective clinical leaders and to empower themselves and their organisations, midwives need to discover and utilise certain philosophies that underpin midwifery in relation to the women and families they care for. That is, a midwife who successfully empowers women could, as a leader, have the capability of empowering his or her followers. Chapter 2 debates this theory in more detail, and Chapter 3 gives some examples from local case studies.

There are midwives in successful leadership positions influencing services at local, national and international levels, from academic and strategic positions (for example, see Chapter 4).

What does this mean for midwifery?

Leadership characteristics, traits and philosophies have been briefly outlined above, but how does this relate to the progression and expansion of midwifery leadership? The early 'trait' theories of leadership that suggest leaders have inborn qualities, rather than acquired skills, could be related to some midwifery leaders who possess a natural ability to lead others. It could be argued, however, that those midwives 'learnt' the skill by working closely with positive role models, which would conform with the views of Handy (1993), who firmly believed in the influence of others on the leadership role.

Theories such as those based on 'situational contingency' describe particular characteristics for dealing with situations, and 'style' theory relates to what the leader actually does. In the complexity of maternity care, it could be suggested that midwives need to utilise some aspects of each of these theories. This would reflect the need to be flexible and responsive to changing situations, and to accommodate the fact that actions may need to change from time to time according to a particular situation.

Historically, midwifery leadership followed the health service model of authoritarian 'top-down' approaches to leading services. Curtis *et al.* (2006) have elaborated on the effects of institutionalised bullying in maternity care, as a reason for midwives leaving the profession. Whilst there may be occasions when it is necessary for midwifery leaders to assume responsibility and make decisions without consultation, a democratic style of leadership may be more acceptable. Pashley (1988) suggests that transactional leadership, described as a process of mutual influence and coalition building, is important for midwives, as they are required to work in partnership with an array of other professionals. In a metasynthesis of the qualitative literature relating to the 'good' leader, Byrom and Downe (2010) note that the traits associated with such leaders could be described as transformational. It could be suggested that leadership traits and characteristics might usefully be identified within individual midwives and then nurtured, supported and developed accordingly.

Developing midwifery leadership: planning for the future

The World Health Organization (2009) suggests that leaders are born with certain personality traits, but they can develop a range of skills to be more effective. In the UK, the Department of Health (2009c) directs the development of leadership capabilities in the midwifery workforce as a high priority. The report proposes that midwives should be given full access to relevant new and existing development opportunities within the NHS and higher education, as they will need to show evidence that they have achieved appropriate preparation for specific roles. A commitment has been made to work with the midwifery profession to develop leadership capacity and enhance quality (DH 2009b).

The Health Foundation (2009a,b) believes that healthcare leaders need to be equipped with a range of skills and competencies to help them meet the wide-ranging challenges within the NHS and has commissioned research to clarify the key, effective interventions to create leadership knowledge, behaviours, skills, competences or 'habits of mind' relating to quality improvement. The study provides the basis for the Foundation's programmes now used to develop leadership capacity (Anderson *et al.* 2009).

In the past there have been several specific leadership development programmes for midwives, particularly for strategic positions such as consultant midwives and heads of midwifery (for example, the Midwifery Leadership Programme developed by the NHS Leadership

Centre). Other courses have been generic development opportunities such as the Leading an Empowered Organisation and the RCN Clinical Leadership programmes, which targeted all NHS staff in mid-senior roles, including midwives.

The aim of the UK government's Leadership Centre (DH 2009d) is to promote leadership development through identifying the role of all leaders in the NHS as one of improving patient care and experience, promoting a healthy population, enhancing the reputation of the NHS as a well-managed and accountable organisation, and finally motivating and developing staff. The Centre provides human resources advice in relation to leadership development and is a useful resource for NHS organisations. However, the process of becoming a midwifery 'leader' is varied and inconsistent. In the past, it was considered appropriate to 'earn' the role through years of experience, rather than gaining a leadership position on merit. Although this may still be the case in some organisations, there is a move towards encouraging those with potential and enthusiasm to lead, with appropriate experience as a basis. So how are midwifery leaders identified and nurtured and given appropriate skills?

In her study, Kay (2007) considered the experience of leadership in a community midwifery service. Recommendations following data analysis included a suggestion that the service must determine what it wants, needs or expects of its leaders. This followed confusion amongst the study participants about what was required of effective leadership in their role.

> I don't know what you want my role to be. You are telling me I am a team leader and you are saying I should be leading things and when I have – for example, I tried to set up a project group, because to me that is very clearly defined within my role ... and my manager said that that wasn't my role and was really angry with me.
>
> (Kay 2007, p.2)

Another recommendation was to consider the qualities existing and aspiring leaders possess and to revise job descriptions, explicitly shaping and defining the role in the community context. The study suggested that the role should be positively promoted and a mentor system for aspiring leaders should be put in place so that development can be supported and encouraged. Kay argued that a career pathway for midwives interested in leadership roles should be developed but maintained that this could involve culture change. This followed the supposition made by one of the participants that:

> ... midwives see their point of registration as the end of the course and that's that. Whereas if you look at obstetricians and the medical profession, when they qualify that is not the end – they are then on

a new career pathway but midwifery or probably nursing don't take that view and it can't go on like that.

(Kay 2007, p.2)

The suggestion is made that in the process of developing leadership capacity within the maternity service, the knowledge and skills needed to meet the demands of any midwifery leadership role should be outlined. The service should consider the experience leaders bring to the post and identify any gaps which may exist between the leader's current capabilities and the requirements of the role.

Jorgensen (2006) proposes that the Knowledge and Skills Framework (KSF) framework currently used within the NHS helps to identifying the skills and knowledge needed by an individual to do their job. Kay (2007) developed a model of determining competency for the leadership role at the level of the midwifery team leader (Figure 1.2). Following identification, Kay (2007) then suggests that a pre-leadership programme for aspiring midwifery leaders and further development training for existing leaders could be considered alongside the KSF.

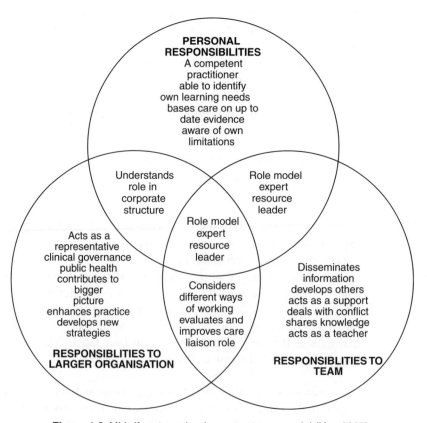

Figure 1.2 Midwifery team leader competency model (Kay 2007).

Community leadership and maternity care

Woman-centred care and transformational leadership philosophies include the use of the words 'empower', 'trust', 'facilitate' and 'mutual respect'. The same words are used to describe community development, a process that gives communities greater control over the conditions that affect their lives through building confidence to tackle problems. Within the NHS, community development approaches to care are more congruent with health visiting services as part of the public health agenda, yet the concept fits well with childbirth philosophy. Maternity care that promotes and supports meaningful relationships between mothers, midwives, obstetricians and other care workers maximises the potential for the health and well-being of the mother, baby and wider family. There is evidence that when an empowering, facilitative approach is taken to providing care, where the mother and family are central to decisions and part of the journey, they are more likely to feel confident with child-rearing and even to become community leaders (Garrod & Byrom 2007; Walsh & Byrom 2009; Byrom & Gaudion 2009). Peer support networks, where mothers support mothers (such as breastfeeding support groups), are an example of this concept. There is an increasing number of user-led pressure groups, appealing for support on the internet and social networking sites, and aiming to improve maternity care through challenging strategic decisions. Service user chairs of groups such as Maternity Services Liaison Committees are an illustration of community leadership that aims to promote and support local maternity services. Chapter 3 provides examples of several midwives who are successfully leading services, and also a mother who began her career through links with maternity services and is now head of policy at the UK's National Childbirth Trust.

The concept of community development not only enhances midwifery leadership but also supports the process of continuously improving maternity services and, more importantly, raises the potential for improved maternal and infant health.

Conclusion

Although a lack of midwifery leadership has been identified, there is a growing body of knowledge in relation to what matters to mothers, midwives and obstetricians and a recognised importance of effective and positive leadership in maternity care. It is also apparent that, as midwives strive for improvements in maternity service, and as they face challenges in doing so, they must aim not only to recognise their own leadership capabilities but also to identify and follow positive role models to help them. Within the UK, opportunities are available to develop leadership capabilities, and, although not all are related to midwifery, the fundamental principles will assist in the move to expand the body of midwifery leaders.

References

Anderson L, Malby B, Mervyn K, Thorpe R (2009) The Health Foundation's position statement on effective leadership development interventions. London, Health Foundation.

Antrobus S, Kitson AA (1999) Nursing leadership: influencing and shaping health policy and nursing practice. *Journal of Advanced Nursing* 29:746–53.

Bass BM (1990) *Bass and Stodgill's Handbook of Leadership Theory, Research and Managerial Applications.* New York, Free Press.

Bednash G (2003) Developing leadership. In Marquis B, Huston C (eds) *Leadership Roles and Management Functions in Nursing: Theory and Application.* Philadelphia, Lippincott, Williams and Wilkins.

Burns JM (1978) *Leadership.* New York, Harper and Row.

Byrom S, Downe S (2010) 'She sort of shines': midwives accounts of 'good' midwifery and 'good' leadership. *Midwifery* 26(1): 126–37.

Byrom S, Gaudion A (2009) Empowering mothers: strengthening the future. In Byrom S, Edwards G, Bick D (eds) *Essential Midwifery Practice: Postnatal Care.* London, Blackwell Publishing.

Cabinet Office (2009) Nominating someone for an honour. www.direct.gov.uk/en/Governmentcitizensandrights/UKgovernment/Honoursawardsandmedals/DG_067917 (accessed June, 2010).

Care Quality Commission (2006) Investigation into 10 maternal deaths at, or following delivery at, Northwick Park Hospital, North West London Hospitals NHS Trust, between April 2002 and April 2005. www.cqc.org.uk/_db/_documents/Northwick_tagged.pdf (accessed June, 2010).

Care Quality Commission (2008) Towards better births: a review of maternity services in England. www.cqc.org.uk/publications.cfm?fde_id=625 (accessed June, 2010).

Christian SL, Norman IJ (1998) Clinical leadership in nursing development units. *Journal of Advanced Nursing* 27:108–16.

Coggins J (2005) Strengthening midwifery leadership. *Midwives* 8(7): 310–13.

Conger JA, Kanungo RN (1994) Charismatic leadership in organisations: the perceived behavioural attributes and their measurement. *Journal of Organisational Behaviour* 15:439–52.

Cook MJ (2001) The renaissance of clinical leadership. *International Nursing Review* 48:38–46.

Curtis P, Ball L, Kirkham M (2006) Bullying and horizontal violence: cultural or individual phenomena? *British Journal of Midwifery* 14(4): 218–21.

Davidhizar R (1993) Leading with charisma. *Journal of Advanced Nursing* 18:675–9.

Dawson S, Garside P, Hudson R, Bicknell C (2009) The design and establishment of the Leadership Council. www.dh.gov.uk/prod_consum_dh/groups/dh_digitalassets/documents/digitalasset/dh_093388.pdf (accessed June, 2010).

Department of Health (2009a) National Leadership Council. www.dh.gov.uk/en/Publicationsandstatistics/Publications/DH_093342 (accessed June, 2010).

Department of Health (2009b) *A High Quality Workforce: NHS Next Stage Review.* London, Department of Health.

Department of Health (2009c) *Delivering High Quality Midwifery Care: The Priorities, Opportunities and Challenges for Midwives.* London, Department of Health.

Department of Health (2009d) Leadership Centre. http://webarchive.nationalarchives.gov.uk/ + /www.dh.gov.uk/en/Managingyourorganisation/Humanresourcesandtraining/Modelcareer/DH_4080689 (accessed June, 2010).

Donnison J (1988) *Midwives and Medical Men: A History of the Struggle for the Control of Childbirth*, 2nd edn. London, Historical Publications.

Garrod D, Byrom S (2007) The midwifery public health agenda; setting the scene. In Edwards G, Byrom S (eds) *Essential Midwifery Practice: Public Health.* London, Blackwell Publishing.

Gould D, Kelly D, Goldstone L, Maidwell A (2001) The changing needs of clinical nurse managers: exploring issues for continuing professional development. *Journal of Advanced Nursing* 34(1): 7–17.

Handy C (1993) *Understanding Organisations.* London, Penguin.

Health Foundation (2009a) Leadership. www.health.org.uk/topics/leadership.html (accessed June, 2010).

Health Foundation (2009b) Improvement Leadership Update. www.health.org.uk/publications/briefings_leaflets/leadership_update.html (accessed June, 2010).

Helgesen S (1990) *The Female Advantage: Women's Ways of Leadership.* Vienna, Women in Management.

International Confederation of Midwives (2010) Introduction to the Young Midwifery Leadership Programme. www.internationalmidwives.org/Projects/YoungMidwiferyLeadershipProgramme/tabid/334/Default.aspx (accessed June, 2010).

Jorgensen F (2006) *What Do You Know About the KSF?* Cambridge, Career Progression Team, Cambridge University Teaching Hospitals NHS Foundation Trust.

Kay L (2007) 'Leading other midwives.' A critical ethnographic inquiry exploring the experience of midwife team leaders. MST (Master of Studies in Primary and Community Care). Cambridge, Cambridge University.

King's Fund (2008) *Safe Births: Everybody's Business. An Independent Inquiry into the Safety of Maternity Services in England.* London, King's Fund.

Kouzes JM Posner BZ (2007) *The Leadership Challenge*, 4th edn. San Francisco, Jossey Bass.

Lewin K, Lippit R, White RK (1990) Theories and styles of leadership. In Bernhard LA, Walsh M (1990) *Leadership: The Key to the Professionalization of Nursing*, 2nd edn. Philadelphia, Mosby.

Mullins LJ (2009) *Management and Organisational Behaviour*, 8th edn. London, Prentice Hall.

National Health Service (2009) NHS Leadership Awards. www.nhsleadershipawards.nhs.uk/ (accessed June, 2010).

Pashley G (1998) Management and leadership in midwifery: part 1. *British Journal of Midwifery* 6:460–4.

Ralston R (2005) Transformational leadership: leading the way for midwives in the 21st century. *RCM Midwives Journal* 8:34–7.

Reinertsen JL, Bisognano M, Pugh MD (2008) *Seven Leadership Leverage Points for Organization-Level Improvement in Health Care*, 2nd edn. IHI Innovation Series White Paper. Cambridge, MA, Institute for Healthcare Improvement. www.IHI.org (accessed June, 2010).

Schein E (2004) *Organizational Culture and Leadership*, 3rd edn. San Francisco, Jossey Bass.

Stanley D (2004) Clinical leaders in paediatric nursing: a pilot study. *Paediatric Nursing* 16(3): 39–42.

Tack A (1984) *Motivational Leadership*. Aldershot, Gower.

Trent BA (2003) Leadership myths. *Reflections on Nursing Leadership* 29:8–9.

Van Maurik J (2001) *Writers on Leadership*. London, Penguin Books.

Vroom VH, Jago AG (1988) *The New Leadership: Managing Participation in Organizations*. New Jersey, Prentice Hall.

Vroom VH, Jago AG (2007) The role of the situation in leadership. *American Psychologist* 62(1): 17–24.

Vroom VH, Yetten PW (1973) *Leadership and Decision Making*. Pittsburgh, PA, University of Pittsburgh Press.

Walsh D, Byrom S (2009) *Birth Stories for the Soul: Tales from Women, Families and Childbirth Professionals*. London, Quay Books.

West MA (2004) *Effective Teamwork: Practical Lessons from Organizational Research*, 2nd edn. Oxford, Blackwell Publishing.

World Health Organization, Partnership for Maternal Newborn and Child Health (2008) *Successful Leadership: Country Actions for Maternal, Newborn and Child Health*. Geneva, World Health Organization.

World Health Organization (2009) Leadership in health promotion: complexity, innovation and closing the gap of implementation (course notes). Melbourne, Australia, Swiss School of Public Health, in collaboration with La Trobe University, School of Public Health and World Health Organization.

Chapter 2
Transformational Leadership and Midwifery: A Nested Narrative Review

Sheena Byrom, Anna Byrom and Soo Downe

Introduction

Examination of the literature on leadership and that relating to midwifery reveals some evolutionary similarities. The dominant theories in both areas appear to be moving away from hierarchical models and towards those based on relationship. In the case of leadership, this has led to a concentration on transformational philosophies, in contrast to earlier approaches based on command and control. In midwifery, woman-centred care has become the ideology of choice, theoretically replacing hierarchies built on professional power bases.

As noted in Chapter 1, leadership theories originally evolved from a rationalist emphasis on objectivity, control, competition and power (Ajimal 1985; Alkhafaji 2001). Research and development in this area in much of the last century used the tools of the rational scientific method (Lewin 1938; Yukl 1989; Barker 1994; Barker & Young 1994; Moiden 2002). This resulted in the dominance of patriarchal values and assumptions (Barker & Young 1994). Following the mechanistic view of science adopted at the time, organisations were viewed as machines (Plsek & Wilson 2001). More recently, a number of theorists in the field, including Barker (1994), have promoted a new view of the world that accentuates human relationships and acknowledges uncertainty. This turn has been termed 'transformational leadership'. It calls for responsive ways of leading, with an emphasis on (so-called) feminine values and beliefs such as caring, nurturing and intuition, to balance patriarchal values (Barker & Young 1994). Transformational leadership theory

Essential Midwifery Practice: Leadership, Expertise and Collaborative Working, first edition. Edited by Soo Downe, Sheena Byrom and Louise Simpson
Published 2011 by Blackwell Publishing Ltd.
© 2011 Blackwell Publishing Ltd.

is grounded in the philosophy that humans are often intuitive and emotional rather than rational, and the belief that scientific methods do not supply answers to all of life's complexities (Davidhizar 1993; George 2000).

A number of authors have claimed a similar history for childbirth (Wagner 1986; Donnison 1988; Oakley 1989; Arms 1994; Bryar 1995; Martin 2001). This interpretation notes the patriarchal effect of medicine on childbirth, and critiques the impact of consequent mechanistic scientific rational approaches on childbearing women and their babies (Peel Report 1970; Roberts 1983; Cahill 2001). In theory, at least, the woman-centred doctrine of the Winterton (DH 1992) and *Changing Childbirth* (DH 1993) reports provided a challenge to this dominant way of seeing. The more recent National Service Framework for Children, Young People and Maternity Services (DH 2004) and *Maternity Matters* document repeat this challenge. Those promoting concepts such as humanistic birth (Davis-Floyd 1991) propose holistic approaches that parallel some of the developments in leadership theory.

Background to concepts of leadership

There are multiple approaches to understanding leadership (Burns 1978; Bennis & Nanus 1985; Bass & 1992; Handy 1993; Kouzes & Posner 1995; Heifetz & Laurie 1997; Mullins 1999; Clegg 2000). The topic has been the subject of comment from distinguished writers from both nursing and midwifery backgrounds (Rafferty 1993; Barker 1994; Page 1995; Kirkham 1996; Hurst 1997; Kirkham & Perkins 1997; Pashley 1998; Fisher & Davidhizar 1998; Kirkham 1999; Ralston 2005).

In the traditional paradigm set out above, leaders have valued characteristics related to authority, control, competition and logic (Davidhizar 1993; Barker 1994). The 'industrial' model frames the construct of leadership within a supervisor/subordinate relationship (Yammarino 1995). Post-Industrial Revolution organisations, including healthcare systems, were built on these beliefs, with the resulting creation of hierarchical structures underpinned by rational and logical decision making (Cottingham 1994). This leadership philosophy was grounded on the theory of positional power (Handy 1993). Van Vugt *et al.* (2004) found that such autocratic leadership styles have a destabilising influence on group members, and that they were not suitable to influence effective change.

In contrast to this approach, Barker (1994, p.82) claims that, due to centuries of experience and the discovery of ambiguous, uncertain elements in the world that humans cannot control, a new paradigm is emerging. Barker and Young (1994) argue that today's leader needs a philosophy rather than a theory of leadership. This philosophical approach is the basis of much of the current literature on transformational leadership.

Transformational leadership and healthcare

Transformational leadership, first described by Burns in 1978, is an emerging philosophy for modern management (Davidhizar 1993; Carless 1998). It stands in direct contrast to a modernist, autocratic, hierarchical style. Its intention is to communicate positive self-esteem and a focus on people (Davidhizar 1993).

There is a plethora of literature on transformational leadership (Burns 1978; Conger & Kanungo 1988; Bass & Avolio 1992; Barker 1994; Kouzes & Posner 1995; Carless 1998; Pielstick 1998; Ralston 2005). It has received more empirical scrutiny in the organisational science literature than have all other leadership theories for the past two decades (Judge & Bono 2000; Lowe & Gardner 2000). Burns (1978) described it as a vibrant style, where leaders connect with followers in such a way as to stimulate a feeling of elevation by the followers, who often then become more active and even become leaders themselves. Although transformational leadership is seen by some to be grounded in moral philosophy (Barker 1994), concrete practical strategies have also been proposed for its development (Pielstick 1988; Bennis 1989; Bass & Avolio 1994; Kouzes & Posner 1995).

Burns (1978) differentiates between transactional and transformational leadership styles. Transactional leadership occurs when one person takes the initiative in making contact with others for the purpose of making an exchange (Broome 1990; Conger & Kanungo 1994). Bass and Avolio (1992) suggest that transformational leadership styles build on transactional theories by broadening the effects of the leader on effort and performance, and they propose that the same leader may display both types of leadership. They also, however, refer to research data which, they claim, demonstrate that transformational leaders are more effective than purely transactional leaders regardless of how 'effectiveness' has been defined or measured.

Kernick (2001), in acknowledging that the health service is a complex environment, supports a change from transactional to transformational styles in this context. Along with others (Marriner-Tomey 1993; Davidhizar 1993; Fisher & Davidhizar 1998; Durnham-Taylor 2000), he believes that transformational leadership theory provides a useful tool for leadership within health and social care, and for effective nurse leadership in modern healthcare settings. Indeed, Davidhizar (1993) claims that the techniques of transformational leadership are a positive response to unrest and dissatisfaction in the healthcare environment. Following a review of UK nursing leadership literature, however, Crook (2001) found that transactional leadership was the predominant style, a style which relies mainly on standard forms of inducement, reward, punishment and sanction by leaders to control followers (Gronn 1997).

The focus of this chapter

Midwives and midwifery have always claimed that they champion a holistic approach to childbirth. It seems logical, then, that transformational leadership may be a natural approach for midwifery leaders. However, despite this apparent synergy, there appears to be little in the literature about the possibility of adopting transformational leadership approaches in midwifery. In order to assess this, a systematic search of the literature was undertaken in an attempt to identify any papers which had explored correlations between the philosophies of woman-centred midwifery care and transformational leadership theory. In the absence of any findings, two purposive narrative reviews were undertaken, in the areas of 'transformational leadership' and 'woman-centred care'. This chapter discusses the methodological approach we developed for the former review, reports the findings, and identifies possible future research in this area. We do not claim that it isinclusive of all the published output in this area. However, we do claim that it captures some of the main themes arising in both research and opinion-based publications related to the nature of transformational leadership.

Methods and findings

Initial systematic search (phase 1)

Although our initial search did not yield any papers which met all our inclusion criteria, the papers we went on to explore in the narrative review were generated by the search. The strategy therefore forms the framework for our review. For this reason, we have set out the details of the strategy below.

Search strategy

The following search terms were used either singly or in combination: *leadership, transformational leadership, nursing, midwife, midwifery.* The following electronic databases and search engines were utilised:

* Premedline and Medline 1966 to September 2009
* CINAHL 1982 to September week 4 2009

Table 2.1   Inclusion and exclusion criteria

Inclusion criteria	Exclusion criteria
Types of study Systematic reviews Research papers (all methods) Expert opinion	*Types of study* Letters to editor Languages other than English

Focus of study
Studies/papers testing or exploring
   possible correlations between
   transformational leadership and
   midwifery philosophies
Studies/papers testing or exploring
   possible correlations between
   transformational leadership and
   nursing philosophies
	Focus of study
	Studies/papers where no connection
	   was made between two philosophies

- AMED 1985 to September 2009
- MIDIRS (The Midwifery Research Database) to September 2009
- Cochrane Database of Systematic Reviews third quarter 2009
- Emerald
- www.findarticle.com.

Reference lists from these sources were also followed up. In order to scope the field as widely as possible, expert opinion and evidence-based work were included alongside controlled and qualitative empirical studies.

This search was initially undertaken in 2002, and subsequently updated to December 2004 and then to September 2009. Inclusion and exclusion criteria are given in Table 2.1.

Findings (phase 1)

No papers were located which fulfilled the requirement that both leadership and midwifery should be the subject of the study. However, in the process of reviewing studies to determine if they met the inclusion criteria, it was noted that the work of three authors turned up regularly in reference lists (Bass 1985; Podsakoff *et al.* 1990; Kouzes & Posner 1995), and that a meta-ethnography of transformational leadership had been published (Pielstick 1998).

Nested review (phase 2)

The decision was made to synthesise the data arising from these index studies, and then to recontextualise ('nest') the resulting themes in a pragmatic narrative summary of the wider literature on transformational leadership. This process was undertaken to generate hypotheses for future studies in the light of a specific contemporary leadership theory, rather than to provide a definitive concept analysis or a systematic review of leadership in general.

Method

The nature and quality of the four index studies were summarised (Table 2.1). The key themes arising from the papers identified in the initial review were summarised, and then synthesised thematically by two of the authors (SB and SD) independently after the first and second searches and then checked against newly emerging literature by AB in 2009. Agreement on the final synthesis was reached by consensus (Table 2.2). We then returned to the wider literature identified in the phase 1 review and organised it against these themes, to see if they were parsimonious and sufficient in describing the underlying philosophies in this body of literature. In formal terms, we were assessing the degree of data saturation that these themes represented. We also consciously searched for disconfirming data. We have termed this process 'nesting'.

Results

The index papers are summarised in Table 2.2. All the studies were undertaken by authors based in the USA. They comprise two multi-method multi-study projects (Bass 1985; Kouzes & Posner 1995), one questionnaire survey (Podsakoff *et al.* 1990) and a meta-ethnography of transformational leadership (Pielstick 1998). The primary themes in each study and the four synthesised meta-themes are presented in Table 2.3. We were able to organise ('nest') all the other literature we had located against these four themes, although some took a negative position. The following sections summarise this literature against our primary themes.

Communicating a vision

Vision has become a very fashionable word in leadership literature (Barker 1994, p.84). Kouzes and Posner (1995) believe that every organisation and social movement begins with a vision, and that it is this force that invents the future. Leaders provide the vision to stimulate energy which accomplishes higher levels of performance and development (Bass & Avolio 1992). Hater and Bass (1988) proclaim that transformational leaders arouse in their followers high performance and new ways of thinking by transmitting a sense of mission. The transformational leader pushes back boundaries and explores new territories, and translates vision into reality by action (Wright 1996). Barker and Young (1994) describe how transformational leaders are value brokers; they concern themselves with values by providing a vision for the future that is exciting yet feasible, and that provides meaning and purpose for all involved. Barker (1994) reflects on Burns' definition of transformational leadership where the essential ingredient is held to be collective purpose. To stimulate an organisation towards its goal, a realistic, credible, optimistic vision must be shared (Barker 1994, p.84). Pielstick (1998) describes several characteristics of a shared vision including inspiration, excitement, motivation and a meaning for all employees and stakeholders.

Transformational leaders are held to be capable of translating intention into reality through communicating their vision and gaining support (Bennis 1982; Conger 1991). Conger (1991) notes the importance of the leader's ability to not only detect opportunities but to describe them in ways which will maximise their significance. Indeed, he claims that crafting and communicating an inspirational vision are critical to the success of the transformational leader. He goes on to offer a detailed explanation of how this can be done through the 'language of leadership' and suggests that it is a critical skill that can be learned. He demonstrates how leaders, through their choice of words, values and beliefs, can craft commitment and confidence in their company missions. For Conger, the leader's words have their greatest impact as symbols, metaphors and analogies that all appeal to the emotions and ideals of followers. Pielstick (1998) also holds that a skilled leader inspires and encourages followers to act through appropriate language, sometimes through the use of emotional appeals and a sense of drama. Such leaders tend to describe changes as opportunities, possibilities or potentialities. They also engage in a mutual sharing of the moral purpose of the vision, and they use this to build relationships.

A transformational leader is at the centre of a socially constructed network allowing a vision to emerge from interaction and dialogue (Kernick 2002). Interaction is crucial; at the operational level, Cottingham (1994, p.90) proposes the use of open-ended questions in transformational leadership. For Pielstick (1998), listening constitutes the most important component of communication for transformational leaders. Indeed, compared to routine work, innovation requires more listening and communication (Kouzes & Posner 1995, p.144). These authors suggest that active listening is a source of inspiration as the

Table 2.2 Summary of included studies

Author	Topic	Design of study	Setting	Sampling strategy	n	Analytic strategy	Comments
Bass 1985 USA	Study of transformational and transactional leadership styles resulting in the Multifactor Leadership Questionnaire	1 Open-ended survey: respondents asked to describe someone who fitted a predetermined description of a transformational leader 2 Sorting exercise, where statements from (1) and from literature review were sorted into 'transformation', 'transactional' or don't know 3 Survey questionnaires containing the 73 data items resulting from (2) 4 'Additional small and large scale studies...' testing these findings	1 US industry 2 US educational institution 3 US army 4 Various	1 Convenience sampling of senior industrial executives 2 Graduate MBA and social science students studying leadership 3 Senior US army officers 4 Educational administrators, world-class leaders, business, government, industrial employees	1 70 2 11 3 104: less than 2% female 4 n varies by study	1 Apparently thematic 2 Descriptive statistical 3 Multivariate and factor analysis 4 Including technical directors, world-class leaders, professionals, educational administrators and industrial managers	This series of work resulted in the widely used Multifactor Leadership Questionnaire (MLQ). This has both transformational and transactional leadership characteristics. The former are included in the analysis in Table 2.2 The work appears to have been rigorous and wide-ranging: however, most of it was undertaken in the US, so there is a risk that it is context specific

Source	Focus	Method	Context	Sample	Analysis	Comments
Podsakoff et al. 1990 USA	Transformational leadership behaviours	Questionnaire survey, designed on the basis of an in-depth prior literature review, followed by q sort analysis by experts in the field Questionnaires given out personally, returned in prepaid envelopes	Multi-national petrochemical company	Sample was 'exempt' employees. Not clear if all eligible employees included	n = 988 Response rate 80% 90% male 95% based in US, Canada or Europe Mean age 40 yrs 53% managers 81.4% college degree 61% belonged to a professional organisation	Confirmatory factor analysis to establish factor structure	There were large correlations for the items on the emerging factors The authors note that the results could be a product of the beliefs and experiences of managers/professionals This study appears to be well designed, if focused on a narrow group of employees
Kouzes & Posner 1995 USA	Results of research into exemplary leadership, resulting in the Leadership Practices Inventory	1 Qualitative open-ended interview survey and open-ended interviews, based on descriptions of leader situations when at personal best	1-4 'private and public sector organisations' 5. Various private, public and voluntary organisations	'Ordinary' people asked to describe extraordinary situations Not clear how the participants were selected	1-4 middle and senior managers 1 n=38 2 n=550 3 n=780 4 n=42 initially, by 1997 n=300	1, 4 ?Content and thematic analysis (not specifically described, but can be inferred from the text) 2, 3, 5 'Psychometric processes', including factor analysis, and reliability and validation	This book reports on research undertaken initially 20 years ago, and continuously updated since The scale development was rigorous, and testing has continued over two decades, and in a wide variety of contexts

(continued)

Table 2.2 (Continued)

Author	Topic	Design of study	Setting	Sampling strategy	n	Analytic strategy	Comments
		2 Survey based on findings of (1) 3 Shorter form of questionnaire based on findings of (2) 4 In-depth interviews to contextualise (3) (1–4 occurred between 1985 and 1987) 5 Eventual output of 1–4 resulted in Leadership Practices Inventory (LPI) then tested between 1987 and 1995 with 'thousands' of additional cases			5 n = approx 60,000 leaders of community, students, church, government and 'others in non-managerial positions'	testing, cross-cultural and discriminate analysis	
Pielstick 1998 USA	Transformational leadership	Systematic 'meta-ethnographic' review	N/A	Details not given	Number of initial hits and of studies included not given	Explained in great detail. Studies were initially ordered into 9 groups. The grouped literature was	Though this is termed meta-ethnography, it appeared to include studies that were not ethnographies. The author states that

| Wang & Huang 2009 Taiwan | Study of the relationship of transformational leadership and group cohesiveness and emotional intelligence | 23 small-medium textile businesses in Taiwan | Measures: 1 emotional intelligence was measured using a 16 self-report items instrument – 5-point Likert scale. Developed by Wong & Law 2002 2 transformational leadership was measured using the 20-item Multifactor Leadership Questionnaire (Bass & Avolio 1997) | Leaders and subordinates sampled Inclusion criteria: 1 each leader had to have 2 or more subordinates rate his/her leadership behaviour 2 at least 2 of the subordinates who completed the leadership measure had to report on their departmental cohesiveness | 51 leaders 252 subordinates Mean age of leaders – 45.2 years Gender – 82% male 12.9 years of company tenure | 1 Hierarchical regression analyses were used to test the hypothesis 2 Descriptive statistical | then analysed using constant comparative analysis aided by Ethnograph. Techniques included open and axial coding of the text of the included papers using open coding | the quality of the included papers was assessed, but there are no tables giving either the characteristics or quality of the included studies. The analysis of the included studies was very rigorous |

(continued)

Table 2.2 (Continued)

Author	Topic	Design of study	Setting	Sampling strategy	n	Analytic strategy	Comments
		3 group cohesiveness was measured by the 8-item tool developed by Dobbins & Zaccaro (1986)		3 the leaders themselves had to complete the emotional intelligence measure Mean age of leaders – 45.2 years Gender – 82% male 12.9 years of company tenure			

Table 2.3 Transformational leadership behaviours: a synthesis of selected papers

Author	Themes	Synthesis of themes
Bass 1985 US	• Charismatic leadership • Individualised consideration • Intellectual stimulation	
Podsakoff *et al.* 1990 USA	• Identify and articulate a vision • Provide an appropriate model • Foster acceptance of group goals • High performance expectations • Provide individualised support • Recognise accomplishments • Intellectual stimulation • Others	✠ Communicating a vision ✠ Building relationships
Kouzes & Posner 1995 USA	• Modelling the way • Inspiring a shared vision • Enabling others to act • Challenging the process • Encouraging the heart	✠ Facilitation through caring ✠ Charisma
Pielstick 1998 USA	• Creating a shared vision • Communicating the vision • Building relationships • Developing a supporting culture • Guiding implementation • Exhibiting character • Achieving results	

leader discovers the new and creative ideas of others. Listening is half of giving feedback (Cottingham 1994), and listening can be a learning opportunity. In this way, communication of a vision can be a reciprocal process for a transformational leader.

Building relationships

Cottingham (1994) proposes that transformational leadership builds on a human need for meaning and that his approach creates leaders who manage with the heart as well as the head. Building relationships reflects the interactive, mutual and shared nature of transforming leader behaviours (Pielstick 1998). From his meta-ethnography, Pielstick noted that transformational leadership behaviour involves being friendly and informal. Such leaders tend to fully engage with followers and treat them as equals when giving advice and offering help and support. Furthermore, these leaders are sincere, personable, helpful, caring and build trust through caring actions (Pielstick 1998). People can only be and act their best in an environment of trust. Establishing and maintaining both organisational and personal trust with others represents the fundamental strategy of the transformational leader (Barker & Young 1994; Barker 1994).

Transformational leaders actively develop relationships with their co-workers, who become more active, motivated and inspired to the extent that the meaning of their work is transformed (Burns 1978). The process is immune to cultural differences and is universally applicable (Bass 1997). Cottingham (1994) asserts that transformational leaders should be visible and friendly, listening to views as they do so, in an attempt to let workers know they have an important contribution to make. Giving feedback is also deemed an important attribute (Cottingham 1994), with recognition of good work done.

Barker claims that transformational leadership cannot exist unless there is organisational trust. In turn, the transformational leader must trust others as a first step in building organisational trust. This virtuous circle can then result in positive relationships between individuals and groups, leading to creativity and innovation (Barker 1994, p.85). In this way, transformational leaders build businesses, or an enterprise such as a healthcare environment, as they build relationships of trust.

Facilitation through caring

Barker and Young (1994) utilise the analogy of a web, in which the transformational leader is the centre, facilitating the flow of information back and forth and making the necessary connection between leader and follower. This then has the potential to generate co-operation and mutual respect, promoting both organisational and individual trust. As the centre of the web, transformational leaders concern themselves with meeting the needs and motivation of followers directly. Barker and Young go on to maintain that, within postmodern organisations, the two most important needs are self-esteem and self-actualisation.

According to a number of authors, transformational leaders facilitate, guide and coach whilst providing encouragement for personal and professional development (Pielstick 1998; Cottingham 1994; Barker & Young 1994; Judge *et al.* 2002; Mancheno-Smoak *et al.* 2009). Paradoxically, Pielstick claims, on the basis of his meta-ethnography, that the role is also seen as that of a servant leader, with leaders serving their followers (Pielstick 1998). Wright (1996) also touches on the possibilities of 'leader as a servant' in the development of others and the realisation of their potential and the facilitation their growth. This entails knowing when to lead from the front and knowing when to fall back to let others lead, empowering them in the process.

This process is based on positive interpersonal relationships. According to Barker and Young (1994), caring is an essential ingredient for a postmodern organisation, and they propose that successful transformational leaders care for, respect and value their followers. In addition, transformational leaders help followers to understand their own values and needs through probing, questioning, debating, talking and listening (Barker & Young 1994).

Charisma

One dictionary definition of charisma is *'the capacity to inspire followers with devotion and enthusiasm'* (Sykes 1976). In the management literature, it is a quality that is believed to empower and facilitate co-operation, creativity and innovation (Davidhizar 1993; Conger 1999). A number of authors have sought to describe it more fully (Bass 1985; Conger & Kanungo 1994; Gronn 1997; Pielstick 1998). Despite the lack of an agreed definition in the management literature, some authors hold that transformational leaders actively see charismatic qualities in their work. This stimulates followers to solve problems in their own way, to the extent that they become capable of leading themselves (Gronn 1997; Bono & Anderson 2005). In doing this, leaders use their idealised influence (charisma) to move followers from concerns of existence to concerns for achievement (Bass 1992; Avolio *et al.* 2004).

However, Pielstick (1998) concludes from his meta-ethnography that charisma arouses controversy amongst transformational leaders. Although some argue that it is a fundamental component in optimising transformation, others maintain that it is a quality only attributed to a leader by a follower. It is worth noting that charismatic leadership styles can also backfire, when followers are neurotically bound (Davidhizar 1993). Indeed, in his investigation of transformational leadership among UK managers, Lim (1997) discovered that little importance was given to charisma, and it was viewed as superfluous to effective leadership.

There is a consensus opinion that an essential trait of a successful leader is having high self-regard and positive self-esteem (Barker 1994; Barker & Young 1994; Pielstick 1998; Bommer *et al.* 2004; Mancheno-Smoak *et al.* 2009). Pielstick (1998) discovered that this was the single most referenced character trait in his meta-ethnography. His data also indicated that transformational leaders have a need for power but use it for empowering others, rather than for their own purposes. In their earlier work, Barker and Young (1994) maintain that transformational leaders have high self-esteem as well as the ability to build the self-esteem of others. It may be that the charismatic impression given by effective leaders is a consequence of these characteristics, rather than an attribute in itself. Despite this, giving a charismatic impression is clearly seen to be important by a number of writers in the field.

Discussion

Barker (1994, p.82) has suggested that nursing services are moving towards decentralisation as opposed to centralisation, from power to empowerment, directive decision making to participatory management and from managerial governance to self-governance. Leaders are increasingly asked to act strategically in a complex and shifting healthcare environment (Mancheno-Smoak *et al.* 2009; Wylie & Gallagher 2009). Strategic planning is a search for meaning in a transforming situation, with strategies based on purposes and goals that are shared between leader, employees and the organisation (Cottingham 1994; Cronshaw & McCulloch 2008). This phenomenon affects midwifery as much as any other healthcare group.

The index papers were all written by authors based in America. This may be seen as a delimiting factor in the wider application of our findings. However, the nesting exercise has indicated that the core themes arising from these index papers have resonance in the wider literature in this area. For this reason, we believe that these themes can act as hypotheses for future research in this area in the context of maternity care. This may be both in terms of formal midwifery leadership, and also in personal leadership on a day-to-day basis. The communication of a vision, building relationships, facilitation through caring, and charisma may also be factors which influence good midwifery care. It is apparent that both the midwife and the transformational leader need effective, interactive communication skills, with a particular focus on listening. Transformational leaders are innovative and charismatic in an attempt to inspire and motivate followers. In the same way, midwives are encouraged to think laterally and work in new ways to meet the needs of clients and maximise the opportunity for a positive birth experience. In order to impart an effective vision transformational leaders must be clear about their own values and beliefs, and they must build relationships based on mutual dignity and respect. These characteristics are also essential for midwives if they are to deliver woman-centred care.

From a theoretical perspective, transformational leadership has been closely linked to so-called feminine traits of listening, valuing others, empathy and emotional intelligence (Bass & Avolio 1994; Barker & Young 1994; Goleman 1996; Bowles & Bowles 1999; Wang & Huang 2009). While this may have been seen as a disadvantage under patriarchal systems of leadership, the impact of feminism has led some sectors of the business world to begin to revalue such traits. These are also important aspects of good midwifery care, whatever the gender of the midwife. This suggests that adoption of transformational leadership styles may be welcomed, at least in some midwifery settings.

This review is clearly limited in that it took a narrative rather than a classically systematic approach to the secondary review. In addition, the selection of the index cases was pragmatic rather than systematic. The concept of 'nesting' literature beyond the index studies arose iteratively during the process of the review, as a way of increasing the validity and reliability of a classic narrative review. We do not claim, therefore, that the review presents the sum total of all the evidence in the area of transformational leadership. We offer the method here for consideration and future development, in the context of reviews which would benefit from consideration of expert opinion and theoretical discussion alongside research papers.

Conclusion

Despite the limitations we have noted in this chapter, we believe that our findings may provide a basis for hypothesising about the nature of transformational leadership and its possible application to midwifery at a number of levels. It provides a framework for the development of qualitative research in this area, and it may act as a basis for future wider-reaching quantitative studies. It may also provide some insights into the nature of and potential for transformational leadership for practitioners, and for managers of midwifery care.

References

Ajimal KS (1985) Force field analysis: a framework for strategic thinking. *Long Range Planning* 18(5): 55–60.

Alkhafaji AF (2001) *Corporate Transformation and Restructuring: A Strategic Approach*. Westport, CT: Quorum Books.

Arms S (1994) *Immaculate Deception II: Myth, Magic and Birth*. Berkeley, CA, Celestial Arts.

Avolio BJ, Zhu W, Koh W, Bhatia P (2004) Transformational leadership and organisational commitment: mediating role of psychological empowerment role and moderating role of structural distance. *Journal of Organisational Behaviour* 25:951–68.

Barker AM (1994) An emerging leadership paradigm: transformational leadership. In Hein EC, Nicholson MJ (eds) *Contemporary Leadership Behavior: Selected Readings*, 4th edn. Philadelphia, J B Lippincott.

Barker AM, Young CE (1994) Transformational leadership: the feminist connection in post-modern organisations. *Holistic Nursing Practice* 9(1): 16–25.

Bass BM (1985) *Leadership and Performance Beyond Expectations*. New York, Free Press.

Bass BM (1997) Does the transactional-transformational leadership paradigm transcend organisational and national boundaries? *American Psychologist* 52:130–9.

Bass BM, Avolio BJ (1992) Developing transformational leadership: 1992 and beyond. *Journal of European Industrial Training* 14(5): 21–7.

Bass BM, Avolio BJ (1994) Shatter the glass ceiling: women may make better managers. *Human Resource Management* 33:549–60.

Bass BM, Avolio BJ (1997) *Full range of leadership development: manual for the multifactor leadership questionnaire.* Palo Alto, CA, Mind Garden.

Bennis W (1982) Leadership: transforming vision into action. *Industry Week* 213 (5):54–6.

Bennis WG (1989) Managing the dream: leadership in the 21st century. *Journal of Organisational Change Management* 2(1): 6–10.

Bennis WG, Nanus B (1985) *Leaders: Strategies for Taking Charge.* New York, Harper and Row.

Bommer WH, Rubin RS, Baldwin TT (2004) Setting the stage for the effective leadership: antecedents of transformational leadership behavior. *Leadership Quarterly* 15:195–210.

Bono JE, Anderson MH (2005) The advice and influence networks of transformational leaders. *Journal of Applied Psychology* 90:1306–14.

Bowles N, Bowles A (1999) Transformational leadership. *Nursing Times* (Learning Curve Supplement) 3(8): 2–5.

Broome A (1990) *Managing* Change. London, Macmillan Press.

Bryar RM (1995) *Theory for Midwifery Practice.* London, Macmillan Press.

Burns JM (1978) *Leadership.* New York, Harper and Row.

Cahill HA (2001) Male appropriation and medicalisation of childbirth: an historical analysis. *Journal of Advanced Nursing* 33(3): 334–42.

Carless SA (1998) Gender differences in transformational leadership: an examination of superior, leader, and subordinate perspectives. *Sex Roles: A Journal of Research.* www.findarticles.com (accessed June, 2010).

Clegg A (2000) Leadership: improving the quality of patient care. *Nursing Standard* 14(30): 43–5.

Conger JA (1991) Inspiring others: the language of leadership. *Academy of Management Executive* 5(1).

Conger JA (1999) Charismatic and transformational leadership in organisations: an insider's perspective on these developing streams of research. *Leadership Quaterly* 10:145–79.

Conger J, Kanungo R (1988) Behavioral dimensions of charismatic leadership. In Conger J.A. *et al.* (eds) *Charismatic Leadership: The Elusive Factor in Organizational Effectiveness.* San Francisco, Jossey-Bass.

Conger JA, Kanungo RN (1994) Charismatic leadership in organisations: the perceived behavioural attributes and their measurement. *Journal of Organisational Behaviour* 15:439–52.

Cottingham C (1994) Transformational leadership: a strategy for nursing. In Hein EC, Nicholson MJ (eds) *Contemporary Leadership Behavior: Selected Readings,* 4th edn. Philadelphia, J B Lippincott.

Cronshaw SF, McCulloch AN (2008) Reinstating the Lewinan vision: from force field analysis to organisation field assessment. *Organisation Development Journal* 26(4): 89–102.

Crook MJ (2001) The Renaissance of clinical leadership. *International Nursing* 48:38–46.

Davidhizar R (1993) Leading with charisma. *Journal of Advanced Nursing* 18:675–9.

Davis-Floyd RE (1991) The technocratic, humanistic, and holistic paradigms of childbirth. *International Journal of Gynecology and Obstetrics* 75(suppl 1): S5–S23.

Department of Health (1992) *The Winterton Report: UK House of Commons Report into Maternity Services*. London, HMSO.

Department of Health (1993) *Changing Childbirth. Report of the Expert Maternity Group* (Chair J. Cumberlege), vol. 1. London, HMSO.

Department of Health (2004) *National Service Framework: Children, Young People and Maternity Services*. London, HMSO.

Dobbins GH, Zacaro SJ (1986) The effects of group cohesion and leader behavior on subordinate satisfaction. *Group and Organization Management* 11(3): 203–19.

Donnison J (1988) *Midwives and Medical Men: A History of the Struggle for the Control of Childbirth*, 2nd edn. London, Historical Publications.

Durnham-Taylor J (2000) Nurse executive transformational leadership found in participative organisations. *Journal of Nursing Administration* 30(5): 241–50.

Fisher L, Davidhizar R (1998) Every nurse is a leader. *Journal of Practical Nursing* 48(2): 16–19.

George J (2000) Emotions and leadership: the role of emotional intelligence. *Human Relations* 53:1027–55.

Goleman D (1996) *Emotional Intelligence: Why It Can Matter More Than IQ*. London, Bloomsbury Publishing.

Gronn P (1997) Leading for learning: organisational transformation and the formation of leaders. *Journal of Management Development* 16(4): 274–83.

Handy C (1993) *Understanding Organisations*, 4th edn. London, Penguin Books.

Hater JJ, Bass BM (1988) Superiors' evaluations and subordinates' perceptions of transformational and transactional leadership. *Journal of Applied Psychology* 73(4): 695–703.

Heifetz RA, Laurie DL (1997) The work of leadership. *Harvard Business Review* January-February: 124–34.

Hurst K (1997) *A Review of the Nursing Leadership Literature*. Leeds, Nuffield Institute, University of Leeds.

Judge TA, Bono JE (2000) Five-factor model of personality and transformational leadership. *Journal of Psychology* 85(5): 751–65.

Judge T, Bono J, Ilies R, Gerhardt M (2002) Personality and leadership: a qualitative and quantitative review. *Journal of Applied Psychology* 87:765–80.

Kernick D (2001) Complexity and healthcare organisation. In Sweeney K, Griffiths F (eds) *Complexity and Healthcare: An Introduction*. Oxford, Radcliffe Medical Press.

Kirkham M (1996) Professionalisation past and present: with women or with the powers that be? In Kroll D (ed) *Midwifery Care for the Future: Meeting the Challenge.* London, Baillière Tindall, 164–201.

Kirkham M (1999) The culture of midwifery in the National Health Service in England. *Journal of Advanced Nursing* 30(3): 732–9.

Kirkham M, Perkins ER (1997) *Reflections on Midwifery.* London, Baillière Tindall.

Kouzes JM, Posner BZ (1995) *The Leadership Challenge: How to Keep Getting Extraordinary Things Done in Organisations.* London, Jossey-Bass.

Lewin K (1938) *The Conceptual Representation and The Measurement of Psychological Forces.* Durham, NC, Duke University Press.

Lim B (1997) Transformational leadership in the UK management culture. *Leadership and Organisation Journal* 18(6): 283–9.

Lowe KB, Gardner WL (2000) Ten years of the *Leadership Quarterly*: contributions and challenges for the furture. *Leadership Quarterly* 11(4): 459–514.

Mancheno-Smoak L, Endres G, Polak R, Athanasaw Y (2009) The individual cultural values and job satisfaction and the transformational leader. *Organisation Development Journal* 27(3): 9–21.

Marriner-Tomey A (1993) *Transformational Leadership in Nursing.* St Louis, MO, Mosby Year Book.

Martin E (2001) *The Woman in the Body: A Cultural Analysis of Reproduction.* Boston, MA, Beacon Press.

Moiden N (2002) Evolution of leadership in nursing. *Nursing Management* 9(7): 20–1.

Mullins LJ (1999) *Management and Organisational Behaviour,* 5th edn. Essex, Prentice Hall.

Oakley A (1989) Who cares for the women? Science versus love. *Nurse/Midwifery Today Midwives Chronicle and Nursing Notes* 102(1218): 214–21.

Page L (1995) Change and power in midwifery. *Birth* 22(4): 227–31.

Pashley G (1998) Management and leadership in midwifery: part 1. *British Journal of Midwifery* 6(7): 460–4.

Peel Report (1970) *Domiciliary Midwifery and Maternity Bed Needs* London, HMSO.

Pielstick CD (1998) The transforming leader: a meta-ethnographic analysis. *Community College Review.* www.findarticles.com (accessed June, 2010).

Plsek PE, Wilson T (2001) Complexity, leadership and management in healthcare organisations. *British Medical Journal* 323:746–9.

Podsakoff PM, Mackenzie SB, Moorman RF, Fetter R (1990) Transformational leader behaviours, and their effects on followers trust in leader satisfaction and organisational citizenship behaviours. *Leadership Quarterly* 1(2): 197–2.

Rafferty AM (1993) *Leading Questions: A Discussion Paper on the Issue of Nurse Leadership.* London, King's Fund.

Ralston R (2005) Transformational leadership: leading the way for midwives in the 21st century. *RCM Midwives Journal* 8(1): 34–7.

Roberts SJ (1983) Oppressed group behaviour: implications for nursing. *Advances in Nursing Science* 5(4): 21–30.

Sykes JB (1976) *The Concise Oxford Dictionary of Current English,* 6th edn. Oxford, Clarendon Press.

Van Vugt M, Jepson S, Hart C et al. (2004) Autocratic leadership dilemmas: a threat to group stability. *Journal of Experimental Social Psychology* 40(1): 1–13.

Wagner MG (1986) Birth and power. In Phaff J (ed) *Perinatal Health Services in Europe: Searching for Better Childbirth.* Geneva, World Health Organization, 195–208.

Wang Y, Huang T (2009) The relationship of transformational leadership with group cohesiveness and emotional intelligence. *Social Behavior and Personality* 37(3): 379–92.

Wong CS, Law KS (2002) The effective leader and follower emotional intelligence on performance and attitude: an exploratory study. *Leadership Quarterly* 12:1502–14.

Wright S (1996) Unlock the leadership potential. *Nursing Management* 3(2): 8–10.

Wylie D, Gallagher H (2009) Transformational leadership behaviours in allied health professions. *Journal of Allied Health* 38(2): 65–74.

Yammarino FJ (1995) Dyadic leadership. *Journal of Leadership Studies* 2(4): 50–74.

Yukl G (1989) Managerial leadership: a review of theory and research. *Journal of Management* 15(2): 251–89.

Chapter 3
What Do Leaders Do to Influence Maternity Services? Midwifery Leadership As Applied to Case Studies

Sheena Byrom, Sue Henry, Mary Newburn, Cathy Warwick and Ngai Fen Cheung

This chapter provides examples of those whose leadership skills have made a difference to midwives, mothers and babies at a local, national and international level. The intention is to increase awareness of leadership skills, to stimulate self-reflection and debate with colleagues, and to share ideas and strategies that enhance midwifery leadership capacity with the aim of improving maternity care.

What is leadership?

Leadership has been described as the 'process of social influence in which one person can enlist the aid and support of others in the accomplishment of a common task' (Chemers 2002), and Chapters 1 and 2 provide a broad overview of the complexities of the subject, in addition to leadership related to midwifery.

The ingredients for successful leadership in general have been debated amongst experts, researchers and philosophers for decades (Burns 197; Kouzes & Posner 2007). There are leadership theories and styles, leadership development programmes, and leadership coaches, yet it appears that the word 'leader' is generally misunderstood and often mistaken for a management role or position of authority.

Essential Midwifery Practice: Leadership, Expertise and Collaborative Working, first edition. Edited by Soo Downe, Sheena Byrom and Louise Simpson
Published 2011 by Blackwell Publishing Ltd.
© 2011 Blackwell Publishing Ltd.

Individuals frequently describe being inspired by leaders, and this may be a family or community leader, professional leader or a political or world leader. Where positive leadership is apparent, shifts in productivity and satisfaction can be remarkable, and research supports the notion that leaders do contribute to key organisational outcomes (Day & Lord 1988; Kaiser *et al.* 2008).

Midwifery leadership

Several midwives have articulated their views of midwifery leadership (Thomas 2005), and others have stressed the importance of developing potential leaders to ensure the profession is able to face challenges within future maternity service provision (Coggins 2005; Ralston 2005). In a phenomenological study, midwives described in detail how good leaders reinforced their confidence and empowered them, which in turn helped them to empower women in their care (Byrom & Downe 2010). The same midwives used terminology which suggested that emotional intelligence (Goleman 1996) was central to their work. This is a concept which has been cited as an important characteristic for successful leadership for the nursing and midwifery profession (McQueen 2004; Hadikin 2006). The use of emotional characteristics when leading others is reiterated by Karen Gulliand (2008), who described the notion that it is a leader's responsibility to keep 'hope' alive. She supports the view of Crammock (2003) that leaders require 'soul', thereby providing a holistic approach to influencing others. This opinion blends well with transformational leadership theory (see Chapter 1 and 2), which is deemed to be suited to female ideal-type leadership styles (Coggins 2005).

Personal experience of observing and being led by a transformational leader shaped and influenced the leadership style of one of the authors (SB). This leader developed and remodelled services through engaging relevant colleagues with personal communication, utilising the skills of others, empowering her team, and taking risks. Positive leadership in action seems to require encouragement and enthusiasm, even in difficult and stressful situations. The case studies that follow illustrate these characteristics, along with a range of other skills and personal qualities.

Case Study 1

Sue Henry is a midwife working in the north west of England as an infant feeding co-ordinator. Sue is passionate about the promotion and support of breastfeeding, and has developed and utilised effective leadership skills evident in the achievement and maintenance of the Baby Friendly Initiative (BFI) accreditation at a hospital trust (two sites) and a primary care trust. In addition, she has led two other services towards accreditation of BFI standards. It is worth noting that the populations served by these healthcare organisations include some of the most socially and economically deprived in the country. Sue's aptitude for 'thinking outside the box' and, more importantly, her ability to encourage and support others to do so has contributed significantly to the success of this work.

Sue: leading local community change, influencing national change

Just recently I have experienced success with a project that realised a personal vision. I have had time to think about the process, and to reflect on the journey from idea to reality. The recognition that I would be or indeed was leading others wasn't a conscious one; it was a process that evolved from beginning to end.

My vision

The idea I had was to find a way to influence local school children's ability to understand breastfeeding and to hold it in their hearts, until they themselves would be making infant feeding choices. From the very start I understood the challenge. I kept forefront in my mind the impact on health outcomes for mothers and babies, and communities at large.

Working within an education system was new for me. Influencing classroom activities would be pushing my boundaries. Listening to local mothers, I learned that, on the whole, students at 16 years were leaving school with no knowledge of breastfeeding. My everyday work involves maximising potential to increase breastfeeding initiation rates, by implementing the Baby Friendly Initiative standards. I was very much aware that we needed to influence all ages to believe in breastfeeding. I had an idea of how this might be achieved. I discussed my plans with members of the North West Breastfeeding Implementation Framework team (North West Regional Public Health Group 2008), who spurred me on with encouragement. I always understood how challenging this project could be, but a personal motto of mine is 'never let go of what you believe in'.

The journey started in January 2007 when I met with Healthy School leads to discuss my vision for embedding breastfeeding education into the school curriculum. I believed it had the potential to make a difference. Rather than simply going in to schools to talk to pupils about breastfeeding, I wanted to use the medium of drama, as it was different, could be fun, and I didn't know of it being done before, so it would be pioneering work. My initial plan was to engage local college students to help me, but I considered that this might be unsustainable as they ended their courses. So I thought it would be good to join with local community mothers, giving them an opportunity to express their voices too, and to develop skills in this work. Together, we would develop a piece of drama that would captivate an audience of 12–13 year olds, and that would ensure they understood about the benefits of breastfeeding. Equally importantly, I wanted to challenge their existing knowledge, their views on breastfeeding in public, and their understanding about the health risks of formula feeding.

I was very fortunate to know a local breastfeeding supporter who was also a skilled actress and who embraced the project idea. Nicky would go on to write the script, and direct the drama to perfection. Also, another two local mothers (and breastfeeding supporters), Amanda and Kirsty, stood out in my mind – and they accepted my invitation to help. As project 'leader', I was myself 'led' by those I asked to help me.

Funding had to be sought to ensure the 'actresses' were reimbursed for their time to develop the piece and to enable us to deliver at least one pilot show. I managed to secure funds from the Primary Care Trust's public health department as the project helped to meet some of their targets such as reducing obesity, promotion of health and well-being and optimum nutrition, health promotion, coronary heart disease prevention and increases in rates of breastfeeding itself.

Learning aims

There was a general commitment for the session to be of excellent quality, and I had great faith in my colleagues whom I had asked to help me achieve this. The learning aim of the session was to provide students with an opportunity to consider breastfeeding as the optimal way to feed babies. We wanted to help students to think about breastfeeding as 'normal', and we wanted them to learn in a way that created interest, through drama. The students would observe this piece of drama, be involved in feedback and discussion, and then offered a handout to reflect on the session.

At the end of the session, the students would understand the health benefits of breastfeeding, the risks of formula feeding, and the environmental implications, and they would be able to consider why mothers may choose or not choose to breastfeed. This would also provide the students with an opportunity to consider how to make breastfeeding more fashionable, and equip them for future informed choices for improved family health.

Early development work

In August 2007 we had the first development time together. I briefed the team about my vision and thoughts for future development. We looked at a draft workbook that would accompany the session, and practical work began. The team had fun with 'voice and room warm-ups', as we explored together our personal thoughts on the benefits of breastfeeding, and possible benefits of formula feeding. This was followed with intense character exploratory work, using character interview style approaches and taking lots of notes along the way. Nicky was to be the 'mum', Amanda the 'boyfriend's mother' and Kirsty the 'pregnant woman'. Scenes were developed and, later, we invited a teenage mother to watch what we had done so far and to share her own ideas and thoughts.

Soon after, a play named 'Sophie's Choice' was born. The play presents a young woman having her first baby. Sophie is receiving information about infant feeding from various sources – her midwife and boyfriend (absent characters), and her mother and her mother in law (staged characters). Sophie does not make her choice during the performance – this is left intentionally open for the students to consider.

School engagement

Letters went out to head teachers, Personal, Social and Health Education (PSHE) leads, the Strategic Director of Children's Services, Healthy Schools leads and other potentially interested individuals and groups. The first school we approached for the pilot was a faith school. We were unsuccessful making a booking as the school governors' board rejected the offer of the drama due to the fact that it could encourage teenage pregnancies and be 'unsuitable' for school children. The school that eventually offered to be a pilot for us was in a socially deprived area of a local town, and the teachers warned us that it may be difficult to captivate the students. They couldn't have been more wrong. The students loved it, laughed with it, and participated in group discussion. This was especially true for the boys. The evaluations were excellent.

Box 3.1   Selected comments from school students following attendance at the first performance of 'sophie's choice'

Boys:

- 'I would choose breastfeeding because it is natural and I would feel good in myself knowing my baby is getting all the nutrients they need'
- 'A big responsibility – make the decision'

Girls:

- 'Thank you for coming to tell us and helping us understand'
- 'I would choose to breastfeed because it will stop my child from becoming ill and prevent me from getting breast cancer'

Comments on the play:

- 'It was a bit unusual/different as we don't usually do stuff like that'
- 'The play was acted very well and made you feel like you want to breastfeed'

Teachers:

- 'Pleasing to see that it wasn't just girls who were engaged'
- 'They'll tell their family. They won't forget it – it will come back to them later. For some it will be the first time they've heard about it'
- 'Actors in-role came across as 'real' characters who gave an effective and believable performance'

Next steps

Initially, it was hard to encourage schools to book the play or even to understand the need for it. However, we received more help financially from the Public Health Department of our local trust, to finance the play in more schools. Another school booked the play, an infant feeding specialist booked it for her 'father's forums' and the team went on to present at a national conference. The North West Breastfeeding Framework Implementation Group were proactive in moving things forward, by encouraging schools via a Healthy Schools link to engage with the play along with the Best Beginnings[1] 'Get Britain Breastfeeding' exhibition[2]. The director of Best Beginnings contacted us and invited the group to write a paper about the aims of the work, which we did. We have since met to pursue opportunities for disseminating the play through all schools in the UK. The vision is now a reality.

One of the group, Amanda, gave me her thoughts on what being involved in the project meant to her.

I was asked by Sue if I would like to be involved in performing a play in schools about breastfeeding. At first I was apprehensive as I had always

[1] www.bestbeginnings.info/
[2] www.getbritainbreastfeeding.org.uk/

suffered massive stage fright and nerves, and was worried that I wouldn't be able to overcome this. But I always want to help Sue, as she has helped me to grow so much, and taught me so much about supporting breastfeeding mums. So I agreed, thinking I would have to work hard to be able to pull this off! I already knew the other people involved, Nicky and Kirsty, as they had been in the local breastfeeding community for a while, we had met at breastfeeding groups and other occasions ...

At the Little Angels conference last year I had to give a talk about my journey from volunteer to paid peer supporter, in front of the whole conference audience, and anyone who saw me do that would say that I shook like leaf and looked about to keel over at any minute. Yet when it came time for us to perform 'Sophie's Choice', in front of the same audience, I just got into it, remembered all my lines and didn't show a bit of my previous terror. On a personal note, being involved with this project has helped me grow tremendously, given me confidence and confirmed that I have some amazing, talented and supportive friends in Sue, Kirsty and Nicky.

With the help of one of the team, Nicky, I felt we reached out beyond the assets of the team we worked with and right to their inner beliefs in themselves. I had to guide them respectfully and give them a strong sense of direction, while keeping the longer term vision clear. The team had to understand themselves and their limitations, but importantly, their ability to develop further.

I don't think you can teach anyone how to lead others, I think you have to work it out for yourself. I feel I learnt special leadership skills by witnessing them from others and exploring my own skills and developing them further. I believe good leaders develop their skills over time and enjoy developing themselves as well as others. Leaders need to be trusted and have excellent two-way communication skills. They have to understand themselves in the first instance, and learn to reflect and improve on a regular basis.

Box 3.2   Top tips for leadership in action

1. Keep learning and learn from your team – develop your 'emotional intelligence'
2. Know your team – they have to want this too – and have plenty of team-time
3. Look out for their well-being – be caring and support them from beneath
4. Keep them informed, as well as other key partners
5. Trust in their own responsibility in the project
6. Ensure everyone understands each other
7. Engage with other partners to support your project
8. Be professional, loyal, and take responsibility

9. Be honest, show courage and have fun
10. Provide direction, influence and commitment, and fill your team with confidence

Community development 'focuses on bringing people together, whilst empowering individuals'. It is associated with the words 'encourage', 'facilitate', 'enable'and 'trust' (Health Development Agency 2004). Midwives have the capability to develop community confidence in improving health locally and in this case, nationally. I feel by handing over the ideas, skills and projects to community members, we will maximise opportunity to build communities and improve health.

And finally, to remember a great and inspirational leader:

We must be the change we want to see in the world.

(Mahatma Gandhi, 1869–1948)

Case Study 2

Mary Newburn is the Head of Policy at the National Childbirth Trust. Mary has used the influences of her mother and of her own childbirth experiences to lead developments within the UK's most popular charity for parents. Mary is well respected and renowned for her expert knowledge in the area of maternity care, and for her natural ability to communicate with women and families, midwives and obstetricians. She also works effectively with politicians, to influence and improve maternity service provision.

Mary: the route to service user leadership

I remember as a little girl being really extremely worried about the prospect of how I could ever give birth to a baby. I was 5 years old when my brother, Hartley, was born. I was very proud of him and pretty much considered him to be mine. Having a baby in the house made a big impression on me – more still the thought of his arrival in the world, and I asked my mum about it.

'Don't worry,' she said, 'You go to the National Childbirth Trust (NCT) antenatal classes and they show you how.' She must have talked to me about labour quite a bit too, because I grew up knowing about pelvic rocking and the benefit for backache labour of kneeling on all fours. Anyway, her response worked for me. She said it with such calm assurance. I had been terrified. If you look down when you're on the loo between your little-girl legs, the prospect of pushing out one of those massive baby heads seems horrific. Yet, I moved on from trepidation to anticipation. The NCT would sort me out.

I think my mum must have talked about having babies and breast-feeding more than was good for me, because I developed an unusual interest in the subject. At 16, I won an award at school and chose Sheila Kitzinger's *Women's Experience of Childbirth* as one of my prize books. It was inserted discreetly between the other two paperbacks on history and literature. Twelve months later I was pregnant and anticipating childbirth for real.

A pregnant teenager, I wasn't perhaps the most likely NCT mum-to-be and I didn't go to classes. My first experience of birth in the 1970s was horrendous. The local 'GP unit' was ruled out when I reached 39 weeks and the baby was still in a posterior position and not engaged. I remember Risedale Maternity Hospital in Barrow as a place of cold white tiles, enema tubes and an irritated house doctor who complained I'd probably be getting her out of bed during the night. The evening, the night and the whole of the next morning stretched out, excruciatingly painful, at times terrifying, achingly lonely and devoid of human comfort and kindness. I was on my own, except for the final stage when a lovely midwife came on duty and said to me 'Come on, we can do it'. For the first time someone had spoken to me directly with warmth and encouragement. Her language joined us together and inspired me. She said 'we' can do it. Her attitude turned the whole experience around for me. She believed in me. And when Gavin was born, face to pubes and looking up at me, he was so amazing. Exquisitely beautiful. And the pain was suddenly over.

The following year, I did go to NCT classes when I was expecting Robin – and I booked a home birth. Again not typical for a woman like me, but my mum had had her four babies at home and really thought you must be absolutely bonkers to think of going near a hospital to have a baby, if you could avoid it.

The 'old school' psychoprophylaxis-style classes were a fantastic help to me. Our teacher in Kendal was a former nurse; she didn't go in for home birth, but she did believe in relaxation and rigorous prep. That time I sailed through the labour, though didn't get the home birth I wanted. Back I went to the Risedale Maternity Hospital in Barrow.

Aged 19 and a childbirth veteran, I then applied to train as an NCT teacher. My friends by this time were working, earning and having fun, or had passed their A levels and gone off to university, so I was wondering what to do with the rest of my life. I really wanted to train as an NCT breastfeeding counsellor as I'd had real difficulties feeding Gavin until I got out of hospital and my mum came to stay. Again, I learned that the strength of her belief, her total confidence in breastfeed-ing and in me was very powerful.

I remember reading the *Infant Feeding Survey* a couple of years later and noting that I had most of the listed characteristics that made me unlikely to breastfeed, including having left school at 16 and being a young mum. Though they'd missed one crucial factor, which is now recognised as highly important: having been around breastfeeding. Having seen my mum and my aunty feeding their babies, it was something I really wanted to do.

Years later, I was so happy to marry Tim and prepare for having another baby. As I thought Lewis might be my last baby and I really wanted to enjoy the pregnancy and birth, I decided to cut and run from the gently disapproving NHS care to an independent midwife who thought I was making sensible, positive decisions in planning a home birth. Lewis, and then Owen, who were both born at home in London in the early 1990s, also taught me a lot about myself, about labour and maternity care. I was older this time, 30 plus, and more experienced. Yet, I met opposition to opting for a home birth which I hadn't when I asked for one in the 1970s in Cumbria. Experiencing just how low-tech birth can be was quite an eye-opener for me. Culturally we have come to believe deep within us that a whole lot of paraphernalia is required to birth a baby safely and most of it most of the time is simply not necessary.

For me, over the course of four births I experienced a growing sense of self-awareness and self-confidence, as well as coming to recognise increasingly clearly how maternity systems constrain women. I was so disempowered the first time. Doped up on pethidine, I was flat on the bed for most of labour and needed the midwife to cut me and pull the baby out. With each of the following births, I was less 'done to', more able to move around and decide what felt right. The fourth time, confident from a previous straightforward home birth, I gave birth standing up, and Tim and I caught Owen together.

So my childhood experiences and my births have been the backdrop to my work and my developing ideas. My mum was a feminist who cared about women's opportunities and who also believed that having babies and breastfeeding were two of the really special things a woman could do in her life. That perspective, the love and excitement shared with Tim of having babies together, and being the mother of four sons makes me both woman centred and passionate about dads being fully part of the whole experience, too.

The stepping stones to my current job are not immediately obvious. Aged 20, I came to London with Gavin and Robin to move back in with my mum. I'd had a really tough few years and felt at quite a low point. I had to get on with life so I enrolled to take some A-levels. Hartley, who was still at home, was a real star. Week after week he looked after my boys while I was at evening classes. Once I moved into a separate flat, I also taught NCT classes for about 12 months to couples who were generally at least 10 years older than I was.

I'd been fortunate to be shown some fascinating anthropology films and to have the chance to take a Sociology GCE while at school. The interest inspired me to apply to read Sociology at the LSE. It was a really tough experience studying for a degree with two young children on a low income, and with quite a bit of emotional baggage to deal with. But I made it through those 3 years and so did Gavin and Robin. I then began work for a PhD afterwards at Essex University on women's relationship careers, but that did get the better of me.

Despite no doctorate, my NCT experience and knowledge of women's health and family issues were the trump cards, I suspect, in landing a job at the NCT as General Secretary elect. It was just a spooky coincidence that when I was looking for a job, that post was advertised. It was a long shot to think I might get it, but taking the chance paid off. The General Secretary role has long since gone, as the NCT roles and responsibilities have been reconfigured several times in the intervening years. Though there have been many changes and the NCT has grown in size and influence, I have always worked on issues of policy, research, parents' involvement in maternity services and lobbying for change.

I feel passionate about women having good preparation and support during labour and birth, the chance to give birth at home or in one of the new birth centres, or in hospital with friendly, kind midwives. I had protracted struggles with breastfeeding, colicky babies and adjusting to the challenges of full-time mothering with badly broken sleep, but I also found feeding and family life enormously special and rewarding. Although I draw on a much wider pool of knowledge and many more parents' stories, the gut-level impact of my own experiences is one of the things that remind me daily of how much it all matters.

Case Study 3

Cathy Warwick is an esteemed midwifery leader and is currently the General Secretary of the UK's professional body for midwifery, the Royal College of Midwives. Cathy has a vast experience of leading others at many levels, including a large London maternity service. Cathy's leadership skills are regularly sought after, and she continues to support the midwifery profession through strategic transformation and change.

Cathy: leading the midwifery profession through inspirational management

King's College Hospital is an acute teaching hospital in south east London. Maternity services are provided to approximately 5500 women each year. The majority of these women experience some degree of social deprivation. The service has a busy obstetric unit, a world-renowned fetal medicine unit and a level 3 medical and surgical neonatal unit. The unit also has a high home birth rate (8%), nine caseloading midwifery practices, and one of the lowest caesarean section rates in London (23.8%).

I took up post at King's in 1993 and worked there in different posts, but always as the lead for maternity services, until leaving in 2008 to become General Secretary of the Royal College of Midwives. During my time at King's I feel we made significant progress towards the provision of women-centred maternity services and in this brief case study I will outline what, on reflection, I see as the key elements of our success.

Most importantly, we had an active vision of what we wanted to achieve. This was women-centred, individualised services for women. The vital word here is 'active'. Without that word, such a vision is simply like motherhood and apple pie. The fact that our vision was active meant that issues such as choice of place of birth, decisions based on risk, and application of guidelines were constantly considered in the light of what women wanted, and not in relation to all of our different professional perspectives and agendas.

Secondly, whilst my leadership was important, responsibility for success was in no way my own. In our complex multilayered, multi-professional NHS, success can never be about an individual. I saw my own role as one of providing a framework for development and winning support for that at a strategic level in the trust and amongst our commissioners. I also had to lead by example, ensuring that motivation remained high, encouraging innovation and, of course, brokering between the inevitability of competing demands and priorities. However, leadership by the whole managerial/clinical team and at all levels in the service was critical. Most developments that took place at King's were as a result of enthusiastic and committed midwives and doctors who saw a way to put our vision into practice. It was the midwives at King's who themselves developed caseloading practices, initiated water birth and supported its introduction into general practice, who led on the development of our midwifery-led guidelines and who challenged our rising caesarean rate.

Two essential components of my role do not always seem to come easily to those running maternity services. Often midwives tell me how their managers show little interest in their ideas and often managers tell me how they cannot foster innovation because of the constraints placed on them by other sectors of their trust, such as the human resources department, or by other professionals who do not seem to believe in home birth or in normalising birth.

Positive leadership is in my view very much about spotting the talented midwives who want to make a difference and being flexible enough and having enough energy to give them the space and opportunity to develop. Of course, some of these midwives may be 'noisy' and 'challenging' but these are the people who will drive services forward and will be most constructive if given a chance. People who want to have a say and who will question what is going on are an asset. The trick is to turn that questioning into something constructive. No one ever said that leadership is easy. In my view, anyone who wants a quiet life will have great difficulty developing services for women.

Effective leadership is also about recognising that service development is not straightforward. It isn't always clear what to do and sometimes new developments entail some kind of risk. A new VBAC (vaginal birth after caesarean section) clinic may have been introduced with the primary outcome of reducing the caesarean section rate. Costs may have been justified on this basis. The audit that accompanied this development may not show this reduction. Perhaps some secondary outcomes such as maternal satisfaction may nonetheless merit the continuation of the new service but, if not, the good leader will have the courage to acknowledge that the change has not worked. Too often, nothing is changed for fear of failure. At King's I believed that 'trying' was vital. Following a cycle of implement, audit and review ensured that we continually modified our approach.

There is a tendency in many big organisations to think about all the reasons why things are not possible, rather than why they are possible. For example, a head of midwifery may be told that the 'rules' will not allow the trust to subcontract a team of independent midwives. I tended to frame my questions to colleagues in human resources or in finance not in terms of 'Can I do this?' but rather 'How can we make this possible?'. Of course, that is not to say that brick walls did not present themselves. The familiar cry of 'There is no money!' rang out just as much at King's as anywhere else. Sometimes we had to acknowledge a setback, but only for the time being. I always held onto the vision, held onto the idea and it was surprising how often a different opportunity presented itself to do the very thing that had once seemed impossible.

It is true that service developments don't always meet with universal support but, too often, the problem is that ideas are shared not at all or too late between one discipline and another. Too often a development is strongly owned by one group but not by another. Successful innovation, successful leadership will most commonly occur when ideas are owned by a wide group. At King's, our home birth service was supported by obstetricians and neonatologists who would, indeed, explicitly refer to it as 'our' home birth service in discussion, suggesting a full engagement in home birth provision. Our midwifery-led guidelines were written by midwives and led by midwives but signed off by the multidisciplinary team. If a service does run into any sort of difficulty, this early attention to getting joint ownership will tend to lead to a 'let's see how we can now work together to minimise this problem' rather than a 'sniping at the idea' approach.

On another tack, service development is often associated with re-configuration or radical overhaul. I never took this approach at King's. I thought it was essential that we recognised the fundamental quality of our maternity service and that it was important not to throw the baby out with the bath water. This meant that we tended to take an evolutionary approach to change rather than a revolutionary one. So often, when managers talk to me about developing home births services, they mention putting all that work in the hands of one small team of midwives, completely ignoring a number of community midwives who may not be doing a lot of home births each year but over the years have helped many women have this choice of birth. Why not let them continue in this way whilst also introducing the new team? Equally, if women start to choose home birth in greater numbers, one team will not be enough so be ready to evolve the next team and the next ...

In addition, whilst recognising the expertise that exists, never underestimate the need for training and development. Each service development, each new initiative needs a component built into the project plan for both off-the-job and on-the-job support. Good leaders will recognise that not all staff embrace change with enthusiasm and that one of the key reasons for this is that they feel nervous and ill prepared. Investment in training and support early on will reap dividends further up the line.

Finally, the biggest challenge of leadership is knowing when to let go. It is hard to develop services and then leave them in the hands of others but, given that this is about teamwork, if you have been truly successful the changes will carry on without you. It is my great delight that since I left King's, two further caseload practices have developed, the business case for a midwifery-led unit has been approved, and the home birth rate has increased and in the last quarter of 2008 was 11.4%.

Case Study 4: leading a cultural change – courage and commitment

Ngai Fen Cheung is a professor and director of the Midwifery Research Unit, Nursing College, Hangzhou Normal University, Hangzhou City, Zhejiang Province, China. Fen has co-lead the development of the first midwifery-led normal birth unit (birthing centre) in China. In order to understand the significance of this achievement, the history and culture of maternity services in China need to be understood. Birth and midwifery in China have always been under the supervision of obstetricians. Since 1952, China has followed the Russian model in midwifery education, in which midwifery in higher education (undergraduate and postgraduate studies) was abolished. Only secondary or vocational education for midwifery has remained since. In China, higher education means a 4-year undergraduate programme after 12 years' education and/or 3 years for postgraduate Master's degree studies, while the secondary education is a 2- or 3-year vocational study and training programme after 9 years compulsory education. The secondary midwifery education was discontinued for a decade beginning in 1966. It has been stopped again since 1993 mainly in the cities. However, the secondary midwifery education has survived in the rural areas (Cheung 2009). Those providing most hands-on maternity care in China are the nursing staff working in the labour room. They consist of a small number of midwives trained before 1993, and those trained through a handful of vocational midwifery colleges or nursing colleges of the universities as nurses 'with a midwifery orientation'.

Since the 1990s, medical interventions and caesarean sections have increased dramatically. Up to 100% caesarean section rates were reported for some units in 2000 (Huang 2000).

Fen is currently teaching research methodology in nursing and midwifery and thesis writing in English to a postgraduate class, supervising Master's degree postgraduate students in their research, and doing midwifery research in China. The research includes an international collaboration in the development and evaluation of the first midwife-led normal birth unit in China, a study on the development of Chinese midwifery, and the development of continuing professional education for Chinese registered midwives in China.

Fen inspired delegates at the Third Normal Birth Conference in Grange in June 2009 with her account of the processes, challenges and outcomes involved in the birth centre development work.

Fen: leading to change – the first midwife-led unit in China

In order to set up a midwife-led normal birth unit (MNBU) in China, I worked out three stages for its development: (1) a structured survey of midwives' views; (2) defining normal birth, the philosophy, management structure and procedures; (3) implementation of the unit. It was a common-sense design. The rationale was that if there was no consensus on MNBU among Chinese midwives in the first place, it was obviously impossible for such a project to start.

The proposal was welcomed by the collaborators after quite a few exchanges of emails and meetings, which could be seen as constructive in our mutual understanding. A multi-tier team led the project. Our chief collaborators in the University of Edinburgh and the nursing college in China provided advice. I was responsible for the ideas, and for direct contact with the head of the hospital midwives to discuss the direction of the project, and to deal with any problems that arose.

Monthly reviews and seminars facilitated our exchange of ideas further. Being inspired, the midwives involved showed a lot of initiatives. As a result, our survey of midwives' views covered not just two hospitals, as originally designed, but six, plus some informal interviews in a further three hospitals in the region. We were able to collect more answers than we planned to have in the satisfaction survey after the project. The key finding was that setting up the birth centre had greatly enhanced midwife–women relationships.

Retrospectively, I have concluded that this was not just the result of a single leader, but of leadership across a team. I may be more of an initiator or possibly an ideologist to stir things up. Once things are set off, I become a co-ordinator to orchestrate the play. The head of the midwives is also in a similar position, only at a different level (I do not think it a hierarchical one) in the project. For my part, I need to have a strong theoretical as well as practical background to join the play. For example, at some stage in initiating the project, some Chinese midwives challenged that the birth centre approach was not new; it was what they always did as midwives. I was able to convince them that while this could be true on some occasions, the birth centre approach was not fundamentally part of midwifery representation, theorising and orientation in China. Perhaps, as we are inspired, we cultivate our subconsciousness, so that this way of doing midwifery becomes more deeply rooted. That is more likely what is required of midwives as practitioners and theorists.

Box 3.3 summarises what has contributed to the success of the MNBU in China. These principles may be transferable to other leadership endeavours elsewhere.

Box 3.3   Key elements for success in leading the move to a birth centre in china

- Understanding the existing birthing care infrastructure to identify the weakness of the existing management
- Close co-operation between midwifery researchers and the educational authorities and hospital authorities to pave the way for midwives' participation in the project
- The mobilisation of midwives' active participation in the project further encouraged the health authority to accept the research for change
- Midwives took the lead in the new management of the birth centre

Discussion

All of these case studies have similarities. They demonstrate the power of transformational leadership in achieving profound change in midwifery practice, philosophies and structures of care delivery.

In her case study, Sue demonstrates transformational leadership traits in her ability to translate her vision to others, encouraging them to believe in her and themselves, and supporting and nurturing them through the process. Throughout Sue's case study, there is a strong focus on building relationships, promoting teamwork and fostering mutual trust. In addition, Sue has recognised the benefits of utilising an empowering model that develops skills within communities, thereby maximising potential to increase social capital (Byrom & Gaudion 2009).

Mary passionately logs her journey to success, and articulately demonstrates a leadership style drawn from family influences and birth experiences, as described in Chapter 1. It could be suggested that Mary had 'inbuilt' leadership characteristics, as demonstrated in her innate determination to succeed, but she also describes several people who influenced her and shaped her future. Mary is now using personal experiences and the influence of others in her everyday work as a leader within the field of maternity care.

Cathy's case study demonstrates her professional courage and a transformational leadership style, where she facilitates innovation and change with a 'can do' attitude. There is a clear description of fostering energy and talent within the workforce, and the empowerment of those who are recognised as having the ability to make a difference. Cathy provides examples of positive approaches to change, and simple leadership strategies that assist in reducing barriers to service development. Involving the multidisciplinary team and encouraging ownership of change and development is a constant message, and her enthusiasm and energy are tangible.

Fen's case study is an example of how effective collaboration and leadership can influence positive change and innovation, even in the most difficult circumstances. Interestingly, Fen uses the analogy of a play when describing the process of change. She recognises talents in others, and describes a 'participative' leadership style. Fen clearly believes that the partnerships and collaboration with specific recognised and influential others were the keys to success. Being a self-defined 'innovator', she was able to develop and articulate her idea, and to mobilise key players to achieve success.

Midwifery leadership needs to expand and gain momentum in an attempt to maximise potential within maternity care services, to promote women- and family-centred care, to increase physiological,

positive birthing, and to encourage and enthuse midwives in supporting the process.

The leaders invited to recount their journeys for this chapter have
provided an insight into how they achieved their vision and ultimate
success. Their skill and capacity to develop others to succeed, and their
influence on maternity service development offer encouragement and
inspiration to all midwives now and in the future.

References

Baby Friendly Initiative. www.babyfriendly.org.uk (accessed June, 2010).

Burns JM (1978) *Leadership*. New York, Harper and Row.

Byrom S, Downe S (2010) 'She sort of shines': midwives' accounts of 'good'
midwifery and 'good' leadership. *Midwifery* 26(1): 126–37.

Byrom S, Gaudion A (2009) Empowering mothers: strengthening the future. In
Byrom S, Edwards G, Bick D (eds) *Essential Midwifery Practice: Postnatal Care*.
Blackwell.

Chemers MM (2002) Cognitive, social, and emotional intelligence of trans-
formational leadership: efficacy and effectiveness. In Riggio RE, Murphy
SE, Pirozzolo FJ (eds) *Multiple Intelligences and Leadership*. Mahwah, NJ,
Lawrence Erlbaum.

Cheung NF (2009) Chinese midwifery: the history and modernity. *Midwifery*
25(3): 228–41. www.elsevier.com/locate/midw (accessed June, 2010).

Coggins J (2005) *Strengthening midwifery. Leadership Midwives* 8(7): 310–13.

Crammock P (2003) *The Dance of Leadership: The Call for Soul in the 21ˢᵗ Century*.
Auckland, New Zealand, Pearson Education NZ Ltd.

Day DV, Lord RG (1988) Executive leadership and organizational performance:
suggestions for a new theory and methodology. *Journal of Management* 14(3):
453–64.

Goleman D (1996) *Emotional Intelligence: Why It Can Matter More Than IQ*.
London, Bloomsbury.

Gulliland K (2008) Leaders and leadership. *Midwifery News* 48: 6, 7.

Hadikin R (2006) Mind the bully: using emotional intelligence. *Practising
Midwife* 9(11): 32–3.

Health Development Agency (2004) *Developing Healthier Communities*. www
.nice.org.uk:80/aboutnice/whoweare/aboutthehda/hdapublications/
hda_publications.jsp?o=538 (accessed June, 2010).

Huang XH (2000) The present and future of Caesarean section. *Journal of Chinese
Applied Obstetrics and Gynaecology* 16(5): 259–61.

Kaiser RB, Hogan R, Bartholomew Craig S (2008) Leadership and the fate of
organizations. *American Psychologist* 63(2): 96–110.

Kouzes J, Posner B (2007) *The Leadership Challenge*. San Francisco, Jossey-Bass.

McQueen A (2004) Emotional intelligence in nursing work. *Journal of Advanced
Nursing* 47:1101–108.

North West Regional Public Health Group (2008) *Addressing Health Inequalities: A North West Breastfeeding Framework for Action.* www.gos.gov.uk/497468/ images/349392/NW_Breastfeeding_Framework_1.pdf (accessed June, 2010).

Ralston R (2005) Transformational leadership: leading the way for midwives in the 21st century. *Midwives* 8(1): 34–7.

Thomas G (2005) Leadership: the undervalued element? *Midwives* 8(10): 425.

Chapter 4
Leadership for Effective Change in Mother and Infant Health: Lessons Learned from a Programme of Work on Breastfeeding

Mary J. Renfrew

Introduction and background

Nutrition in pregnancy, infancy and early childhood has a fundamental contribution to make to health and well-being in the short, medium and long term. Inadequate food and nutrition affect women and children in both developed and less developed countries, and problems are greatest among those already disadvantaged by poverty and inequalities. Inadequate nutrition in pregnancy and infancy can continue to affect the health and well-being of children as they grow up, and can even have an impact on the health of their own subsequent children, resulting in an intergenerational cycle of deprivation and ill health. Tackling this is a major international challenge; improving maternal and child nutrition would help progress towards four out of the eight UN Millennium Development Goals (MDGs: United Nations 2008).

Midwives have a key opportunity to make a positive impact as they are likely to be in close contact with families at this crucial time. However, an important issue is that, for many years, adequate information about nutrition and breastfeeding has not been included in education and training programmes for midwives or other health workers, and core knowledge and skills are lacking. Added to this is

Essential Midwifery Practice: Leadership, Expertise and Collaborative Working,
first edition.   Edited by Soo Downe, Sheena Byrom and Louise Simpson
Published 2011 by Blackwell Publishing Ltd.
© 2011 Blackwell Publishing Ltd.

the fact that many factors affecting food and nutrition are sociocultural-political, involving a complex mix of commercial interests, public attitudes, women's (dis)empowerment, and problems in health service organisation. They are therefore hard for midwives to influence alone.

Since 1997 the Mother and Infant Research Unit (MIRU) has been examining ways to improve the health and well-being of childbearing women and infants. We are a multidisciplinary research unit, established and led by a midwife, conducting research in health and related social care. We listen to women and babies and the professionals who work with them, and draw the links through from evidence to policy and practice. We use our critical analyses of evidence to underpin knowledge-based strategies for change and to inform education. We have developed a programme of work on strategies to address inequalities in health that has included work with families from very low-income backgrounds, teenagers and women from minority ethnic communities; one major focus of this work has been infant and young child feeding.

Our experience has shown us that to make a difference, it is important to start by identifying evidence-based effective strategies that will work in different situations and with diverse groups. It is not enough, however, to identify strategies and expect them to work. Barriers to change need to be recognised and tackled positively. Such barriers include the often unrecognised constraints on women's choices, the fact that particularly vulnerable families are often not reached or even included in studies, a lack of understanding among health workers of cultural differences in the way families live their lives, interprofessional and cross-sectoral divides, and the organisational bureaucracy that can stop the implementation even of changes likely to make a powerful difference. Our experience has also demonstrated that planned change can work, and that critical analysis of evidence, with appropriate expertise and collaboration, underpinned by effective, informed leadership, are essential components of the multifaceted change strategy needed to tackle a complex issue.

In this chapter, breastfeeding will be used as a case study to examine ways of creating change. The scale of the problem will first be outlined, to place it in context internationally and in relation to the work of midwives and others working in maternity care. Ways in which our work has attempted to address the challenges will then be described, drawing out lessons for leadership in creating change at scale.

The model of leadership that we have developed to tackle multifaceted challenges is described. I call this informed, collaborative, sustained leadership as its value is derived from a sound knowledge base, it is only as strong as the collaborations developed with other leaders in their own fields, and it must be sustained over long periods for real change to occur.

The case of infant and young child feeding

The feeding of infants and young children is a particularly complex example of the challenges of maternal and child nutrition. The widespread use of breastmilk substitutes has a fundamental adverse impact on child health and survival. It has been estimated, probably conservatively, that around 1.3 million infants and young children die each year as a result of a lack of appropriate breastfeeding (WHO 2003); many times more than this will suffer ill health and developmental delays in the short, medium and long term. Suboptimal breastfeeding alone is estimated to be responsible for around 1.4 million child deaths and 44 million DALYs[1] annually (Black *et al.* 2008). The use of breastmilk substitutes has a major impact in both industrialised and less developed country settings, with detrimental infant health and development outcomes seen even in developed countries, including increased gastrointestinal disease, lower respiratory tract infection, sudden infant death syndrome, and impaired cognitive development for the infants (e.g. Howie *et al.* 1990; Ip *et al.* 2007; Quigley *et al.* 2007; Kramer *et al.* 2008). It has an impact on the health of the mother too, such as increased breast cancer in premenopausal women and decreased birth spacing in settings where no other form of contraception is available (e.g. Kennedy & Visness 1992; Collaborative Group on Hormonal Factors in Breast Cancer 2002). It is hard to think of any other single intervention that has such a broad and long-lasting impact on health.

Globally, breastfeeding rates, and especially rates of exclusive breastfeeding that result in the biggest health benefits, declined throughout the 20th century, concomitant with the increased availability, affordability and marketing of manufactured alternatives, the increased medicalisation of healthcare, and especially of pregnancy and birth, and the increased employment of women outside the home without suitable arrangements provided for them to continue to breastfeed (Wolf JH 2003, Crowther *et al.* 2009). As a consequence, by the fifth decade of the 20th century breastfeeding rates were very low across developed countries, reaching down to single figures in some communities. Health professionals who trained from the 1950s onwards were exposed to formula feeding as the norm, and there was no training in the basic curriculum for midwives, doctors, neonatal nurses or health visitors to support women to initiate and continue breastfeeding (Dykes 2006).

Paradoxically, rates have become particularly low in poorer communities, where babies had most to benefit from the positive impact of breastfeeding. Although Scandinavia quickly noticed and reacted

[1] DALYs (disability-adjusted life years) are a measure of potential years of life lost and years of productive life lost to disability.

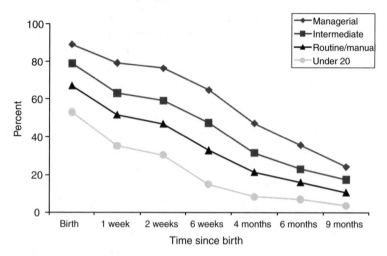

Duration of breastfeeding by mothers' socioeconomic group plus under 20s - 2005

Figure 4.1 Rates of initiation and duration of breastfeeding (partial and exclusive) from birth to 9 months in the UK, for all socio-economic groups and for under 20s. Data derived from Bolling *et al.* 2007.

positively to the decline in rates (Heiberg *et al.* 1995), other developed countries did not, and rates fell and remained low for decades (e.g. Foster *et al.* 1997; Hamlyn *et al.* 2002; Bolling *et al.* 2007). Lowest of all were Ireland, the UK and the US, with young, low-income women in these countries being least likely to start to breastfeed (Figure 4.1). Sadly, these countries have also been among the biggest exporters of aid and healthcare to developing countries, which have in turn been adversely affected by the lack of knowledge and skills among the incoming health workers about infant and young child feeding.

As a consequence, in the first decade of the 21st century, alternatives to breastfeeding, and early weaning, have become embedded as norms in most countries. Those who do start to breastfeed often stop very quickly; 90% of UK women who stop breastfeeding are reported to do so before they want to, with resulting distress (Bolling *et al.* 2007). Even in countries where breastfeeding is the norm, exclusive breastfeeding is becoming less common.

Over the years, breastfeeding has been rendered largely invisible in many developed countries, where it is now rarely seen in public, many women report that it is embarrassing to breastfeed in front of others, and formula feeding has become the normative image of infant feeding (Henderson *et al.* 2000). One study found that teenagers from deprived backgrounds even considered breastfeeding to be 'immoral' (Dyson *et al.* 2010a). The first challenge to creating change in breastfeeding is, therefore, that many people do not believe the lack of breastfeeding to be a problem, including health professionals and even midwives. Some midwives in the UK and internationally have argued that the support of women with breastfeeding is not part of the role of the midwife (personal communication). Some commentators even argue in defence of formula feeding (e.g. Rumbelow 2009). Some health organisations continue to publish adverts for breastmilk substitutes (including the RCM's *Midwives* and the *British Journal of Midwifery*) in which misleading messages are given on the grounds that women need to have a choice and that health professionals need to know about alternatives to breastfeeding, instead of understanding that such advertising promotes misinformation and the impression of equivalence between breastfeeding and its substitutes, and helps to undermine women's choice to breastfeed. Some academics have interpreted the difficulties women describe with breastfeeding as reasons to stop its promotion, instead of tackling the underlying problems (e.g. Lee 2007; Wolf JB 2007). Paradoxically, some feminists see breastfeeding as another mechanism for oppressing women (e.g. Wolf N 2003) instead of seeing women's struggle to breastfeed as a result of the way in which society is shaped by the values of those who do not have the care of children. Even in the face of serious, large-scale public health issues resulting from inadequate formula manufacture, such as the death and illness of hundreds of thousands of babies in China (Parry 2008), the lack of recognition of the damage caused by the use of breastmilk substitutes continues.

The challenge therefore reaches well beyond individual women and the maternity services to public attitudes, the media, commercial interests, advertising and marketing, images and perceptions of sexuality, women's employment, lack of health workers' education and training, and the lack of co-ordinated – or any – policy framework. The issue is multifaceted and fraught with layers of history, emotion, misinformation and guilt (Akre 2006).

The consequence of this is that the burden has fallen disproportionately on individual women and their families, and on individual health workers. Without societal-level change to enable women to breastfeed, women are likely to encounter difficulties such as painful feeding, the baby crying inconsolably, and worries about the baby's weight loss or slow weight gain (Bolling *et al.* 2007). They may face choices about going back to paid employment while finding it hard to continue to breastfeed, and they will find it challenging to feed their babies in public spaces – some even in their own homes (Dyson *et al.* 2010a). The historical lack of good-quality health workers' education and training in this topic means that they may not have the skills and expertise to help (Renfrew *et al.* 2006). Even if they do, the lack of consistent information and support from colleagues may result in their input being ineffective. This in turn is likely to result in a cycle of guilt and blame, and those who advocate breastfeeding being branded as 'zealots' and their knowledge and skills discounted (e.g. Smale 2006).

A major difference between 2010 and the 1960s is that strong evidence is now available of the health catastrophe that has resulted from the use of breastmilk substitutes, and health policy has responded on both global (WHO 2003, Cattaneo 2005, Dykes & Hall Moran 2009) and national (NICE 2008, DH 2009) levels. The important question is: now that the problem has been left to develop for so long, and breastfeeding knowledge and skills have been largely lost by women and health professionals alike, is it possible to reverse the trend?

In summary, this issue is amongst the most challenging of those facing health professionals. It is deep-seated, and it is affected by sociocultural-political factors as well as the clinical circumstances of each woman and her baby. The public, and even many health professionals, do not even recognise that a serious problem exists; the idea of (near enough) equivalence between breastfeeding and artificial substitutes has taken firm hold in the minds of many, so that even gaining consensus on the fact that there is an issue to be addressed is a challenge. It is also evident that if the multifaceted nature of infant feeding can be successfully addressed, lessons will be learned about creating change that could be applied to similarly complex problems such as smoking cessation and reducing interventions in labour.

Creating effective change

Understanding the situation is the first step in addressing it. The preceding analysis is an essential part of the process and underpins all subsequent planning. To then move towards the creation of effective change, co-ordinated work is needed on different levels, tackling the multifaceted issue with effective and consistent action in different sectors. When working with an issue of this complexity, appropriate change cannot be effected by a lone voice or in the absence of evidence.

I have been involved in the field of infant and young child feeding for about three decades, conducting empirical research and reviews, and working for change (see, for example, early work published as Houston, including Houston 1981, 1987; Houston *et al*. 1983, 1984). I established the MIRU in 1997, and since then one of its main themes has been maternal and infant nutrition, including breastfeeding. The team working on this theme, in collaboration with colleagues in different sectors, has identified, developed and worked to implement multifaceted strategies to transform breastfeeding in the UK and internationally. This work on creating change has developed in part as a component of the dissemination of our research work. We also work to integrate our research with education and with policy and practice, and this approach

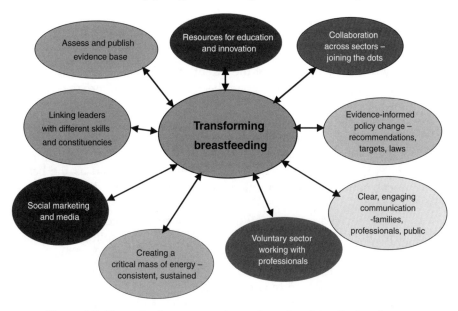

Figure 4.2 Elements of programme to create and sustain effective change.

is an integral component of the programme on maternal and infant nutrition.

Some of the aspects of this programme of work will be described here as an example of the multi-layered approach needed to create complex change at scale. Although the context of much of the work we describe is the UK, we are aware that it has had an impact internationally and has influenced practice and policy with a wide impact in a range of settings.

Figure 4.2 summarises the different dimensions in which our programme of work has sought to influence change. Our experience is that working across all of these fields is essential. Some specific components will be described here.

Critical analysis of the evidence base

Our starting point for creating change has consistently been an examination of the evidence base on what is already known about interventions that will work to tackle the barriers and to enable women to breastfeed. We have conducted a series of critical and systematic reviews which have been widely published and used internationally. They have examined both the initiation and duration of breastfeeding, and include public health and policy as well as clinical interventions (see, for example, Inch & Renfrew 1989; Enkin *et al.* 1995; Sikorski *et al.* 1999, 2003; Renfrew *et al.* 2000, 2005; Fairbank *et al.* 2000; Dyson *et al.* 2005; Britton *et al.* 2007; Moreton *et al.* 2008; Renfrew *et al.* 2009a, 2009b).

These reviews have been published as web-based documents, in books and in peer-reviewed journals, and findings and recommendations have been widely presented at conferences in the UK and internationally. We have evidence of the extent of their reach. For example, over 82,000 copies of one review have been downloaded (Fairbank *et al.* 2000), and another review ranks 27th out of over 5500 Cochrane reviews in terms of the number of times it has been accessed (Britton *et al.* 2007). A review published in September 2009 has been downloaded over 21,300 time in the first 4 months of its publication (Renfrew *et al.* 2009a). We know that these reviews have been used as the basis of local, national and international policy. This will be discussed in later sections.

Our reviews, several of which have been carried out in collaboration with the Centre for Reviews and Dissemination, follow best practice in the conduct of structured and systematic reviews. This includes extensive searches to identify all relevant material, systematic analysis of each included study with independent checking, and ensuring that all recommendations relate to the findings (Centre for Reviews and Dissemination 2008, Higgins & Green 2009). In addition to specific reviews of intervention studies, we have conducted reviews that include a wide range of research approaches where appropriate. We ensure that our reviews of controlled studies of interventions are informed by other relevant research including qualitative studies, and by clinical and public health knowledge and engagement in the field. Our reviews reach beyond a straightforward critique of the methods and findings of studies to a critical analysis of the wider field, and recommendations for future research, policy and practice are informed by what has not yet been done as well as what has. Whenever possible, these reviews also include an inequalities analysis, seeking to identify information – or gaps in information – about the effectiveness of interventions in different population subgroups such as young women or socio-economically deprived families. We recognise that there is unlikely to be one single approach that will work in different settings, and we work to identify characteristics of effective interventions that can be used to inform the design of approaches tailored to fit the needs of local populations.

Our review teams are multidisciplinary and have included midwifery, paediatric, public health, anthropology, physiology, nutrition and breastfeeding expertise as well as methodological expertise in health services research and social science and input from service users. Reviews also have extensive input from advisory groups which include other academics, expert practitioners, policy makers and representatives of childbearing women, to ensure that all relevant perspectives are captured and that the findings and recommendations have the support of an extensive and engaged community.

The importance of this comprehensive and thorough examination of the evidence base cannot be overestimated. It is essential to avoid creating change that would do more harm than good, or that could promulgate ideas that are ineffective and thereby waste goodwill and resources. Through such reviews, knowledge, analysis and critical thinking can be widely disseminated for use in a range of settings, and consistent knowledge can underpin diverse activity.

Creating collaboration across sectors – joining the dots

One of the most far-reaching activities in terms of creating change has been our work to identify ways of implementing effective strategies and overcoming barriers to change. In one influential project that started in 2005, having first identified evidence-based interventions from our reviews, we then conducted a national consultation with practitioners, service user groups, policy makers and managers about how these might work in practice and how barriers to change might be overcome. Using both electronic consultation and structured face-to-face workshops involving over 600 people from diverse sectors, disciplines and levels of seniority, we developed a detailed blueprint for effective change (Renfrew *et al.* 2008; Dyson *et al.* 2006, 2010b). The impact of this work has been profound, and at many levels. Many of the individuals who participated in this process have become informed advocates of evidence-based change. As they included very senior people, the outcome has been to promote the informed and effective leadership needed in different sectors. This has been particularly important in a field where senior people, leaders in their own fields and organisations, are often misinformed about this topic for the reasons outlined above. This work has allowed them to reassess their previous views and to take in new knowledge.

Also important was the way the work was conducted, which respected the input of very junior as well as more senior people from a range of disciplines and across health and social care sectors. It therefore modelled the sort of participation and joint working needed to create change. The publications that resulted from this work have had an impact on documents including the new *World Class Commissioning Guide* (DH 2009), the *Unicef Baby Friendly Initiative Community Review* (Unicef 2008), and the NICE public health guidance on maternal and infant nutrition (NICE 2008). It also formed the basis of the UK Breastfeeding Manifesto (www.breastfeedingmanifesto.org.uk).

The Breastfeeding Manifesto was drawn up in 2006 as a result of recognition that a consistent national approach was needed to create cross-sectoral change, and to implement the effective evidence-based strategies we had identified. The idea was initiated by Alison Baum (who also established Best Beginnings, see below), supported by the MP David Kidney, and was developed and agreed by a core group of 20 organisations, and is now managed by the National Childbirth Trust. It was launched in 2007; since then it has received support from over 35 organisations (see Box 4.1), hundreds of MPs, and many thousands of individual supporters, who together form the Breastfeeding Manifesto Coalition. It has influenced national policy, including the draft Single Equality Bill and work to restrict advertising of breastmilk substitutes. My chairing of the Coalition Steering Group in its first 2 years allowed me the privilege of working closely with outstanding individuals who themselves lead influential organisations. Together, our work helped to establish the organisation and to set the direction of travel. Working with so many organisations with diverse interests and agendas is never straightforward; each has its own agenda and obligations to its membership. Creating a cohesive joint organisation such as the Coalition required a clear focus on the goals of the new organisation, and effective, participatory working practices.

Box 4.1 Members of the breastfeeding manifesto coalition

Association of Breastfeeding Mothers
Baby Feeding Law Group
Baby Milk Action
Best Beginnings
Biological Nurturing
Birthlight
BLISS
Bosom Buddies
Breastfeeding Network
Childfriendly Places
CPHVA
Fatherhood Institute
Friends of the Earth
Independent Midwives Association
La Leche League Great Britain
Lactation Consultants of Great Britain
Little Angels
Maternity Action
MIDIRS
National Childbirth Trust
National Obesity Forum
Royal College of General Practitioners
Royal College of Midwives
Royal College of Nursing

Save the Children UK
The Baby Café Charitable Trust
The British Dietetic Association
The Food Commission
The Royal College of Paediatrics and Child Health
The United Kingdom Association for Milk Banking
Unicef UK
UNISON
WOMB
Women's Environmental Network

At the same time as the Coalition was developing, so was the charity Best Beginnings. This charity has a goal of addressing inequalities in child health and enabling every child to have access to excellent care from the very beginning (www.bestbeginnings.info). It has advocated for evidence-based change and developed key resources to support breastfeeding women. I was privileged to chair the Board in its formative 2 years, and I remain a trustee. Best Beginnings has produced high-quality, evidence-based resources including a DVD now given free to every pregnant woman in the UK ('From Bump to Breastfeeding') and an art exhibition produced by art students that has also resulted in posters that are widely distributed throughout the NHS. The use of media skills and social marketing approaches is a valuable way of giving messages to the public – especially young people – and countering the advertising and marketing of formula milk. The next tranche of work includes a toolkit to support breastfeeding education with young school children, and a DVD for families with babies in neonatal units.

The voluntary sector has been key in the creation of change in infant feeding. The National Childbirth Trust (NCT), La Leche League (LLL), the Breastfeeding Network (BfN) and the Association of Breastfeeding Mothers (ABM) have worked tirelessly to support women and to create change, and it is recognised that their trained counsellors and advisors are better informed than many health professionals (McFadden *et al.* 2006; Renfrew *et al.* 2006). All of the MIRU's work in this field has involved the voluntary organisations in some capacity; voluntary organisations have directly informed our reviews, disseminated our findings, and advocated for evidence-based change. We have worked with the leaders of these organisations – for decades in the case of the NCT – to inform and support each other's work.

One of the challenges is that voluntary sector and health service workers often work separately, yet both groups have a lot to offer. In the light of our very positive working relationship with colleagues in the voluntary sector, we were interested in whether greater joint working would be possible. One of our projects examined whether or not lay workers, trained by a voluntary organisation but without qualifications as a health professional, could work with health professionals to enhance training and improve care (Spiby *et al.* 2003). The project was based in deprived areas in a multiethnic northern city and developed out of our existing engagement with the NHS and related social care across the city. The work involved three lay practitioners working across community, Sure Start, hospital and university settings. The model they used was women centred and evidence based. Activities included teaching health professionals, antenatal education for women and family members, and direct care for women after birth. The project was very positively evaluated, and has been mainstreamed into the PCT and Sure Start services in the city. It has demonstrated that not only is joint working possible, but it can enhance the quality of care and improve the education of health professionals.

In 2004 we were funded by the Health Development Agency (HDA) to lead the new national Public Health Collaborating Centre for Maternal and Child Nutrition. This had two streams of work – one which examined the evidence base and informed public health guidance and one which developed practice. A year later the HDA's work was transferred to NICE and the practice development work was discontinued as a result, but for a year we worked across four health economies in deprived areas of the country to develop networks and a model for whole health economy practice development. We drew on our experiences described above and other work over many years to evolve a model that has now been used by others to inform cross-sectoral working (Renfrew *et al.* 2006). Figure 4.3 shows the stages of the process that we developed, and Box 4.2 outlines the main elements of our conceptual framework. These elements run through much of the work described here, and it seems to be the combination of these aspects that creates the environment in which change is enabled.

Box 4.2 Elements of conceptual framework for practice development (from renfrew *et al.* 2006)

Evidence-based approach

All proposed interventions will be based on a rigorous assessment of the published literature, together with practitioner and user views of that evidence base.

An eclectic mix of approaches and models will be drawn on, based on evidence of 'what works' in different communities.

Multisectoral and multidisciplinary working, including service user/consumer perspectives

Health professionals, other relevant professionals from social and education sectors, community and lay workers, users/consumers and their families will all have a role in informing and delivering the ongoing programme of work.

Mainstreaming and sustainable systems

The programme will work to mainstream maternal and child nutrition into all relevant work programmes of other agencies and organisations, to avoid a sense of being 'initiativebased' and to create sustainable change.

Existing networks and resources will be used wherever possible to ensure an embedded approach to practice development, and to create new systems only when necessary

Solid foundations will be built for long-lasting change and to avoid a 'dash for growth'.

Participatory approach to consultation and communication

All collaborative work will be based on a democratic and participative approach where all constituencies of interest have an equal voice at all stages, regardless of seniority or background.

Work will address all levels of the organisation, i.e. from senior-level policy makers, through regional and local levels, to practitioners in the field, and service users/consumers and their families, and will include approaches at the level of the individual, organisation, service and community.

Embedded evaluation

All approaches used will be evaluated, and findings from these evaluations will be synthesised and widely disseminated to stakeholders, including policy makers and professional leaders, and other appropriate audiences.

Evidence for effective policy making

Change at scale needs effective policy to drive and sustain local, regional and national activity. Our reviews and the national consultation work described above have informed policy including NICE guidance

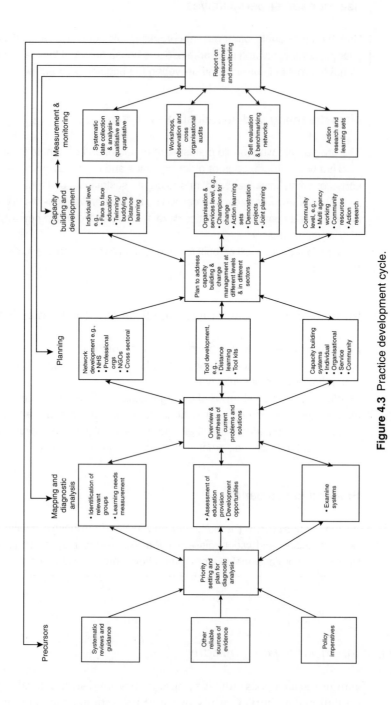

Figure 4.3 Practice development cycle.

(NICE 2008), the Unicef Baby Friendly Initiative Community Review and standards (Unicef BFI 2008), and local hospital policies. An essential component of effective policy making is information about impact. In 2009 we worked with the Department of Health (DH) London and the national Public Health Observatory for Child and Maternal Health (ChiMat www.chimat.org.uk/) to map breastfeeding services across London. The work involved extensive input by the London Breastfeeding Co-ordinator, Francesca Entwistle, and all the London-based infant feeding leads. The aim was to bring together information about breastfeeding rates in individual PCTs and hospital trusts with the services available, to inform commissioners, health professionals and the public as well as policy makers about the availability and impact of breastfeeding services. Using the information gathered, it is also possible to see if services are evidence based, and matched with population need (Dyson *et al.* 2009). Data are available at www.childrensmapping.org. uk/breastfeedinglondon and http://yhpho.york.ac.uk/IADataServer/ MapSelect.asp.

A further resource is being developed to offer women and families the ability to identify their nearest services. Over time, it is planned also to map these data against health outcomes such as gastroenteritis and respiratory tract infection, to examine the longer term impact of service changes. The value of the project was recognised by senior policy makers, and national roll-out started in 2009.

This mapping project has been valuable in several different ways. It has provided novel data about services and rates that give information to local commissioners, providers and families, and this will continue on a national level as the project is rolled out. It also demonstrated the potential contribution of this sort of data collection, collation and dissemination; we now have access to information that can drive service improvement, tailored to the needs of the local population, and this could be done in a similar way for other topics, such as tackling caesarean section or smoking rates. From a leadership perspective, it offers an example of collaborative multidisciplinary working; the leaders in the organisations involved (MIRU, ChiMat, Children's Services Mapping and DH London) each played an invaluable role, and the active involvement of the infant feeding leads across London resulted in very high-quality data.

Clear, engaging communication – families, professionals, public

Much of the spread of the ideas and information described here has resulted from our emphasis on clear and engaging communication, written and verbal. We have worked across the spectrum to communicate with women themselves, health and related professionals from all backgrounds, policy makers, commissioners and the public. This work has included academic papers – some of which have been cited here – books for health professionals (e.g. Renfrew *et al.* 2000), and for women (e.g. Renfrew *et al.* 2004). It has also involved frequent media interviews and well over 100 conference presentations in the UK and 11 other countries in the past ten years. The information given has been derived from complex academic analysis, but we have worked to keep the messages clear, succinct and consistent while avoiding being patronising or simplistic. This work has been crucial to the success of the spread of the messages. Audiences in a wide range of sectors, senior to junior, have heard accurate, consistent and appropriate messages to inform their own work.

Future developments

In 2005 we carried out a national learning needs assessment in which a serious deficit was identified in the education and training of health professionals from all disciplines, but especially medical professionals (McFadden *et al.* 2006; Wallace & Kosmala-Anderson 2007). Although this deficit was known, the scale was striking. The Unicef UK Baby Friendly Initiative (BFI) was already working to address the problem through its accreditation of NHS trusts and staff education. We are now developing a distance learning resource together with Unicef UK BFI for multidisciplinary groups, including doctors, neonatal nurses and support workers, to fill the learning gap and try to ensure that women receive consistent, accurate advice from all health workers. These resources will be available from autumn 2010.

A further new development is our collaboration with the novel Health Innovation and Education Cluster (HIEC), which started work in spring 2010. The aim of this work is to support innovation and improved education, and ultimately to improve outcomes. Our breast-feeding work will be developed within this framework, bringing innovation and change into the mainstream of NHS procedures. We will also develop further initiatives, based on the lessons we have learned from our breastfeeding work, to create change in care in labour and birth, reduce unnecessary interventions and promote normal birth. We recognise the importance of evaluating methods of innovation and change, and this will be built into our work with the HIEC.

Conclusion

As I write this chapter at the start of 2010, it is evident that strategies and activities to enable women to breastfeed are in place across the UK, in community and hospital settings, in health and social care, involving the voluntary sector and support workers as well as health professionals. I have seen examples of effective leadership in local communities, hospital trusts, regional offices, charities, voluntary organisations, professional bodies and universities, involving directors of public health, MPs, NICE, the Department of Health, Unicef UK BFI, service commissioners and managers, individual midwives, peer supporters, health visitors and academics. Similar examples are in place and developing internationally. The networks that have developed are strong, supportive and an outstanding example of how change involving large numbers of people can happen. There is a lot of work still to do. Although data on breastfeeding rates demonstrate that initiation rates are rising consistently, work to support women to continue to breastfeed in a society that is not yet breastfeeding friendly remains critically important, especially in communities where breastfeeding is far from the norm.

Informed, collaborative, sustained leadership for implementation of change at scale

Our work has taught us valuable lessons about leadership, expertise and collaboration that have evolved into a way of working that we believe will be effective in other topic areas.

To contribute to the creation of change at scale, we have found it essential to begin with a critical analysis of the situation. To be effective, such analysis needs an assessment of the evidence base to illuminate the context of the problem and to inform strategies that will work, as well as ways of tackling the barriers.

Close working with organisations and individuals across the country and internationally has been integral to all stages of our work. We have worked with leaders in different fields of activity who have developed consistent messages and strategies in their own fields – social marketing, policy, education and politics as well as health. This combination of perspectives and activity reaches parts of the system that a more unilateral approach would not.

I have observed another outcome to this close working. The reinforcement that occurs as consistent messages come through from different professional and public groups in different settings – a critical mass of consistency and agreement – has resulted in a transformation of perspectives. Work to promote and protect breastfeeding has become mainstream, recognised as a priority (e.g. HM Government 2008), and co-ordinated effortss have developed across the UK and internationally.

The model of leadership that we have developed to tackle multifaceted challenges is not entirely new. It contains elements of transformational leadership such as those discussed in Chapters 1 and

2 (see, for example, Burns 1978; Bass & Avolio 1994), including intellectual stimulation and idealised influence. It is principle centred (Covey 1992), in relation to continual learning, being service oriented, believing in other people and being synergistic. Added to these characteristics are other essential qualities. Our leadership model is grounded in the use of good-quality evidence and is informed by the expertise and experience of others. It is collaborative. It draws together those with different skills, works across sectors and uses a wide range of approaches. It tests out ideas that can then be adopted or modified by others, and disseminates knowledge for others to adapt and implement in their own setting. It influences, informs and links together leaders with different skills and constituencies to work together for a common goal. By working in different ways and different settings, it creates a critical mass of effort and energy to provide impetus and sustain change in the longer term. Over time, it continues to work on the issue of interest, and to give clear and consistent messages, updating those as needed. It looks at the bigger picture and puts in place mechanisms for sustained, system-wide change. It pulls important but neglected problems into view and works to embed solutions in the mainstream of healthcare and the wider society.

It is self-evident that such work depends not on one person but on many, each bringing their contribution, skills, expertise and talents. The main lesson I have learned is that creating change at scale requires not only the confidence to ask others to follow, but the ability to work in collaboration and to follow others in turn. The payback from that approach is the successful implementation of change, and the balanced, respectful and rewarding relationships that result.

Acknowledgements

Our work in the MIRU is based on collaboration and teamwork. I am indebted to all my MIRU colleagues over the past 13 years. In regard to this work in particular, I thank Jenny Brown, Lalitha D'Souza, Lisa Fairbank Dyson, Jo Green, Joyce Marshall, Felicia McCormick, Alison McFadden, Brian McMillan, Mary Smale, Helen Spiby, James Thomas and Mike Woolridge.

A complete list of our knowledgeable, influential, generous and talented external colleagues would not be possible, but our work in the past 12 years would not have had the critical input, energy and reach it has achieved without Jim Akre, Susanne Arms, Sue Ashmore, Rebecca Atchinson, Alison Baum, Rosie Dodds, Janet Calvert, Helen Duncan, Francesca Entwistle, Chloe Fisher, Gill Herbert, Mike Kelly, Belinda Phipps, Amanda Sowden, Louise Wallace, Tony Williams, and the Cochrane Pregnancy and Childbirth Group.

Our work has been funded by sources including the Health Development Agency, National Institute for Health and Clinical Excellence, NHS R&D Programme, National Institute for Health Research, and the Department of Health.

References

Akre J (2006) *The Problem with Breastfeeding*. Amarillo, TX, Hale Publishing.

Bass B, Avolio B (eds) (1994) *Improving Organizational Effectiveness Through Transformational Leadership*. Thousand Oaks, CA, Sage Publications.

Black RE, Allen LH, Bhutta ZA *et al.* for the Maternal and Child Undernutrition Study Group (2008) Maternal and child undernutrition: global and regional exposures and health consequences. *Lancet* 371:243–60.

Bolling K, Grant C, Hamlyn B (2007) Infant Feeding Survey 2005. A Survey Conducted on Behalf of the Information Centre for Health and Social Care and the UK Health Departments by BMRB Social Research. www.ic.nhs .uk/statistics-and-data-collections/health-and-lifestyles-related-surveys/ infant-feeding-survey/infant-feeding-survey-2005 (accessed June, 2010).

Britton C, McCormick F, Renfrew M, Wade A, King S (2007) Support for breastfeeding mothers. *Cochrane Database of Systematic Reviews* 1:CD001141.

Burns J (1978) *Leadership*. New York, Harper and Row.

Cattaneo A (2005) Breastfeeding in Europe: a blueprint for action. *Journal of Public Health* 13:89–96.

Centre for Reviews and Dissemination (2008) Systematic Reviews. CRD's guidance for undertaking reviews in health care. www.york.ac.uk/inst/ crd/systematic_reviews_book.htm (accessed June, 2010).

Collaborative Group on Hormonal Factors in Breast Cancer (2002) Breast cancer and breastfeeding: collaborative reanalysis of individual data from 47 epidemiological studies in 30 countries, including 50302 women with breast cancer and 96973 women without the disease. *Lancet* 360:187–95.

Covey S (1992) *Principle-Centred Leadership*. New York, Simon and Schuster.

Crowther SM, Reynolds LA, Tansey EM (eds) (2009) The Resurgence of Breastfeeding, 1975–2000. Transcript of a Witness Seminar held by the Wellcome Trust Centre for the History of Medicine, London, 24 April 2007. Volume 35.

Department of Health and Department for Children (2009) *Commissioning Local Breastfeeding Support Services*. London, Department of Health.

Dykes FM (2006) *Breastfeeding in Hospital: Midwives, Mothers and the Production Line*. Oxford, Routledge.

Dykes FM, Hall Moran V (2009) *Infant and Young Child Feeding: Challenges to Implementing a Global Strategy*. Oxford, Blackwell.

Dyson L, McCormick FM, Renfrew MJ (2005) Interventions for promoting the initiation of breastfeeding. *Cochrane Database of Systematic Reviews* 2: CD001688.

Dyson L, Renfrew MJ, McFadden A, McCormick F, Herbert G, Thomas J (2006) *Promotion of Breastfeeding Initiation and Duration: Evidence into Practice Briefing.* London, National Institute of Health and Clinical Excellence.

Dyson L, Entwistle F, McCormick F, Renfrew MJ (2009) London Breastfeeding Services Mapping Project. Submitted to DH Regional Public Health Group, London, for web publication in 2010.

Dyson L, Green JM, Renfrew MJ, McMillan B, Woolridge M. (2010a) Factors influencing the infant feeding decision for pregnant teenagers living in urban areas of socio-economic deprivation – the moral dimension. *Birth* 37(2): 141–9.

Dyson L, Renfrew MJ, McFadden A, McCormick F, Herbert G, Thomas J (2010b) Policy and public health recommendations to promote the initiation and duration of breast-feeding in developed country settings. *Public Health Nutrition* 13(1): 137–44. www.nice.org.uk/aboutnice/whoweare/aboutthehda/ hdapublications/hda_publications.jsp?o=738 (accessed June, 2010).

Enkin M, Keirse M, Renfrew MJ, Neilson J (1995) *A Guide to Effective Care in Pregnancy and Childbirth.* Oxford, Oxford University Press.

Fairbank L, Renfrew MJ, Woolridge MW, Sowden A, O'Meara S (2000) Systematic review to evaluate the effectiveness of interventions to promote the uptake of breastfeeding. *Health Technology Assessment* 4(25). www.hta.ac. uk/fullmono/mon425.pdf (accessed June, 2010).

Foster K, Cheesbrough S, Lader D (1997) *Infant Feeding 1995: A Survey of Infant Feeding Practices in the United Kingdom.* London, HMSO.

Hamlyn B, Brooker S, Oleinikova K, Wands S (2002) *Infant Feeding 2000. A survey conducted on behalf of the Department of Health, the Scottish Executive, the National Assembly of Wales and the Department of Health, Social Services and Public Safety in Northern Ireland.* London, Stationery Office.

Heiberg E, Endressen E, Helsing E (1995) Changes in breastfeeding practices in Norwegian maternity wards: national surveys 1973, 1982 and 1991. *Acta Paediatrica* 84:719–24.

Henderson L, Kitzinger J, Green J (2000) Representing infant feeding: content analysis of British media portrayals of bottle feeding and breast feeding. *British Medical Journal* 321:1196–8.

Higgins J, Green S (eds) (2009) *Cochrane Handbook for Systematic Reviews of Interventions Version 5.0.2* (updated September 2009). www.cochrane-handbook.org (accessed June, 2010).

HM Government (2008) *PSA Delivery Agreement 12. Improve the Health and Wellbeing of Children and Young People.* Norwich: Stationery Office.

Houston MJ (1981) Breastfeeding: success or failure? *Journal of Advanced Nursing* 6(6): 447–54.

Houston MJ (1987) Breastfeeding, fertility and child health: a review of international issues. *Journal of Advanced Nursing* 11(1): 35–40.

Houston MJ, Howie PW, Smart L, Mcardle T, McNeilly AS (1983) Factors affecting the duration of breastfeeding. 2 Early feeding practices and social class. *Early Human Development* 8(1): 55–63.

Houston MJ, Howie P, McNeilly A (1984) The effect of extra fluid intake by breastfed babies in hospital on the duration of breastfeeding. *Journal of Reproductive and Infant Psychology* 1:42–8.

Howie PW, Forsyth JS, Ogston SA, Clarke A, Florey CD (1990) Protective effect of breastfeeding against infection. *British Medical Journal* 300:11–16.

Inch S, Renfrew MJ (1989) Common breastfeeding problems. In Chalmers I, Enkin M, Kierse MJNC (eds) *Effective Care in Pregnancy and Childbirth*. Oxford, Oxford University Press.

Ip S, Chung S, Raman G. *et al.* (2007) Breastfeeding and maternal and infant health outcomes in developed countries. *Evid Rep Technol Assess (Full Rep)* 153:1–186.

Kennedy KI, Visness CM (1992) Contraceptive efficacy of lactational amenorrhoea. *Lancet* 339:227–30.

Kramer MS, Aboud F, Mironova E. *et al.* (2008) Breastfeeding and child cognitive development: new evidence from a large randomized trial. *Archives of General Psychiatry* 65:578.

Lee E (2007) Health, morality, and infant feeding: British mothers' experiences of formula milk use in the early weeks. *Sociology of Health and Illness* 29:1075–90.

McFadden A, Renfrew MJ, Dykes F, Burt S (2006) Assessing learning needs for breastfeeding: setting the scene. *Maternal and Child Nutrition* 2:196–203.

Moreton JA, King SE, D'Souza L, McFadden A, McCormick F, Renfrew MJ (2008) *Review 4: The Effectiveness of Public Health Interventions to Promote Safe and Healthy Milk Feeding Practices in Babies*. NICE Maternal and Child Nutrition Programme, 2008. www.nice.org.uk/nicemedia/pdf/MCNReview4Milk Feeding.pdf.

National Institute for Health and Clinical Excellence (2008) *Improving the Nutrition of Pregnant and Breastfeeding Mothers and Children in Low-Income Households*. NICE Public Health Guidance 11. London, NICE. www.nice. org.uk/PH011 (accessed June, 2010).

Parry J (2008) Contaminated infant formula sickens 6200 babies in China. *British Medical Journal* 337:a1738.

Quigley MA, Kelly YJ, Sacker A (2007) Breastfeeding and hospitalization for diarrheal and respiratory infection in the Millennium Cohort Study. *Pediatrics*, 119:e837–e842. www.pediatrics.org/cgi/content/full/119/4/e837 (accessed June, 2010).

Renfrew MJ, Woolridge MW, Ross MGill H (2000) *Enabling Women to Breastfeed. A Review of Practices Which Promote or Inhibit Breastfeeding – With Evidence-Based Guidance for Practice*. London, Stationery Office.

Renfrew MJ, Fisher C, Arms S (2004) *Bestfeeding: How to Breastfeed Your Baby*, 3rd edn.Berkeley, CA, Celestial Arts/Random House.

Renfrew MJ, Dyson L, Wallace L, D'Souza L, McCormick F, Spiby H (2005) *The Effectiveness of Public Health Interventions to Promote the Duration of Breastfeeding: Systematic Review*. London, National Institute of Health and Clinical Excellence. www.nice.org.uk/nicemedia/pdf/Breastfeeding_ vol_1.pdf.

Renfrew MJ, McFadden A, Dykes F. *et al.* (2006) Addressing the learning deficit in breastfeeding: strategies for change. *Maternal and Child Nutrition* 2:239–44.

Renfrew MJ, Dyson L, Herbert G. *et al.* (2008) Developing evidence-based recommendations in public health-incorporating the views of practitioners, service users and user representatives. *Health Expectations* 11:3–15.

Renfrew MJ, Craig D, Dyson L, McCormick F, Rice S, King SE (2009a) Breastfeeding promotion for infants in neonatal units: a systematic review and economic analysis. *Health Technol Assess* 13:40. www.hta.ac.uk/fullmono/mon1340.pdf (accessed June, 2010).

Renfrew MJ, Dyson L, McCormick F. *et al.* (2009b) Breastfeeding promotion for infants in neonatal units – a systematic review and economic analysis. *Health Technol Assess* 13(40): 1–146, iii–iv.

Rumbelow H (2009) Exposing the myths of breastfeeding. *The Times*, July 20th.

Sikorski J, Renfrew MJ, Pindoria S, Wade A (1999) *Support for Breastfeeding Mothers (Cochrane Review)*. Cochrane Library, Issue 1. Oxford, Update Software.

Sikorski J, Renfrew MJ, Pindoria S, Wade A (2003) Support for breastfeeding mothers: a systematic review. *Paediatric and Perinatal Epidemiology* 17:407–17.

Smale M, Renfrew, MJ, Marshall J, Spiby H (2006) Turning policy into practice: more difficult than it seems. The case of breastfeeding education. *Maternal and Child Nutrition* 2:103–13.

Spiby H, Ker R, Smale M, d'Souza L, Renfrew MJ (2003) Introducing a consumer-practitioner into breastfeeding practice. In: Dykes F (ed) *Infant Feeding Initiative: A Report Evaluating the Breastfeeding Practice Projects 1990–2002*. London: Department of Health.

Unicef UK Baby Friendly Initiative (2008) *The Seven Point Plan for Sustaining Breastfeeding in the Community* (revised). London, Unicef UK.

United Nations (2008) The UN Millennium Development Goals (MDGs). www.un.org/millenniumgoals/goals.html (accessed June, 2020).

Wallace LM, Kosmala-Anderson J (2007) Training needs survey of midwives, health visitors and voluntary-sector breastfeeding support staff in England. *Maternal and Child Nutrition* 3:25–39.

Wolf JB (2007) Is breast really best? Risk and total motherhood in the National Breastfeeding Awareness Campaign. *Journal of Health Politics, Policy and Law* 32(4): 595–636.

Wolf JH (2003) Low breastfeeding rates and public health in the United States. *American Journal of Public Health* 93:2000–10.

Wolf N (2003) *Misconceptions: Truth, Lies and the Unexpected on the Journey to Motherhood*. Port Moody, BC, Anchor.

World Health Organization (2003) *Global Strategy for Infant and Young Child Feeding*. Geneva, World Health Organization.

Part II
Expertise
Introduction to Part II

Louise Simpson

Expertise has been cited as an essential component of good-quality care. There are a wide range of theories and scholarly texts that address the nature of expertise. However, it is an elusive phenomenon, with various definitions proposed in the literature. From these definitions, it would appear that both knowledge and experientially based skills are fundamental to expert practice. However, how experts translate this knowledge and experience into expert practice is not immediately evident.

This section consists of four chapters specifically focusing on aspects of expert practice. In Chapter 5, Soo Downe and Louise Simpson aim to explore theories and applications of expertise in general, and in the context of healthcare, specifically in relation to nursing, medicine and midwifery.

They continue their exploration of the issue in Chapter 6, with a focus on expertise in intrapartum midwifery practice. Based on the findings of two studies, a meta-synthesis and a series of group and individual interviews, the chapter focuses on the essential characteristics and skills that facilitate optimal birth outcomes for women, and thus determine expert practice. The rationale, aims, methods and emerging themes are presented first. The rest of the chapter examines the findings in depth, as a basis for developing a theory of midwifery expertise for the future.

In Chapter 7, Denis Walsh describes how expertise and clinical skills can be enhanced through education. Denis explores the concept of expertise against the backdrop of the educational events he has been running for midwives all over the UK and in parts of Europe, Australia and New Zealand. The first part of the chapter is dedicated to the context of maternity care and the rationale for the normal birth workshops, with attitudes and beliefs and the birth environment being the main focus of exploration. The final part of the chapter focuses on the practical aspects of the normal birth workshops, including the content of the sessions, and how midwives have applied them in practice.

As a counterbalance to the emphasis on professional expertise, Anne Davenport presents a series of case studies in Chapter 8. These are built on her experiences in South America and they explore the role of traditional midwives in preserving local and cultural childbirth expertise. Anne explores the enactment of authoritative knowledge in maternity care, and proposes ways in which both traditional and formal midwifery expertise can be valued and used synergistically in practice, to make relationships stronger and to catalyse systems that support healthy, happy, stable mothers, babies and families.

The four chapters in this section present a theoretical and practical exploration of the concept of expertise, with emphasis being placed on intrapartum maternity care.

Chapter 5
The Notion of Expertise

Soo Downe and Louise Simpson

Introduction

Expertise has been cited as an essential component of good-quality care. It would be logical to assume, therefore, that the development and maintenance of clinical expertise would be of interest to health care policymakers and organisations (Hardy *et al.* 2002). However, expertise is an elusive phenomenon (Peden-McAlpine 1999). According to the Longman Online Dictionary[1], an expert may be defined as 'a person who is very knowledgeable about, or skilful in, a particular area'. Other online dictionary sources define experts as 'someone who has a special skill or special knowledge of a subject, gained as a result of training or experience'[2] or 'one whose special knowledge or skill causes him to be regarded as an authority'[3.] From these definitions, it would appear that both knowledge and experientially based skills are fundamental to expert practice. How experts translate this knowledge and experience into expert practice is not immediately evident.

This chapter aims to explore the concept and application of expertise in general, and in the context of healthcare, specifically in relation to nursing, medicine and midwifery.

[1] www.askoxford.com/ (accessed June, 2010)
[2] www.ldoceonline.com/ (accessed June, 2010)
[3] http://dictionary.oed.com (accessed June, 2010)

Essential Midwifery Practice: Leadership, Expertise and Collaborative Working, first edition. Edited by Soo Downe, Sheena Byrom and Louise Simpson
Published 2011 by Blackwell Publishing Ltd.
© 2011 Blackwell Publishing Ltd.

General concepts of expertise

There is a fairly large literature that describes levels of proficiency, across a range of occupations. Researchers in this area have, however, tended to focus on chess players in their studies of how expertise is expressed. Classically, Dreyfus and Dreyfus (1980) studied chess players to explore the progress made from those beginning to play, to those who were consistently successful in tournaments. Based on their data, and on later studies with airline pilots, they proposed five stages of skill acquisition (Box 5.1).

Box 5.1　Five-stage model of skill acquisition (Dreyfus & Dreyfus 1980)

Novice: the beginner is governed by rules and procedures, regardless of context.

Advanced beginner: at this stage, the novice is beginning to pay attention to the general context of their decisions and actions.

Competence: competent practitioners are now in a position to choose a course of action from a range of possibilities. They are able to take responsibility for their decisions.

Proficiency: the proficient practitioner becomes emotionally involved in their practice and, therefore, learns from positive and negative experiences. They can see beyond rules to goals. However, their actions are still fundamentally based on rules and operational procedures.

Expertise: experts swiftly identify what is needed and how to achieve this. Based on the extensive experiences they have at their command, experts respond in a manner that is so rapid and accurate that it seems to be intuitive. Dreyfus argues that experts do not appear to think, calculate responses or solve problems. They 'do what normally works' (Dreyfus & Dreyfus 1986, p.30).

While there appears to be fairly general agreement that individuals develop in stages towards becoming experts, there is disagreement about how they might do this. The influential work of Ericsson and colleagues (Ericsson & Smith 1991a; Ericsson 1996) proposes, and demonstrates, that experts in a range of disciplines (including chess playing, dance and medicine) don't become so by chance. Ericsson's work builds on the idea of the so-called '10-year rule', which suggests that those who become technical experts only do so after a minimum of 10 years of focused practice. Again, this was first proposed in relation to expertise development among chess players (Simon & Chase 1973) and later generalized to other domains (Bloom 1985; Ericsson *et al.* 1993; Howe 1999). In this analysis, expert practice explicitly does not emerge as a consequence of normal everyday work but as a result of deliberate, extra effort that is fully directed at the particular domain in which expertise is sought.

A range of theorists subscribe to this view, and they have further demonstrated that this kind of expertise has a very narrow application. They argue that those who are experts are not automatically more intelligent, faster or stronger than those who are not experts, and those who are naturally gifted will not become experts unless they engage in deliberate, focused practice over a long period of time. They also argue that experts are usually not able to transfer their capacities from one domain to another – that is, expertise is domain specific. Ericsson is a leader in this field, working with colleagues to assess the nature of expertise based on a series of scientific experiments that are reliable, reproducible under laboratory conditions, and measured in absolute terms. This may be possible to do for physical skills that are clearly circumscribed and relatively invariant, such as playing an instrument or even performing certain surgical procedures. It is more difficult to see how such experiments can be designed to assess expertise in the complex and multifactorial contexts of teachers, yachtsmen or health-care workers who are working in unpredictable situations, such as accident and emergency departments or labour wards.

Some authors in this field take a more nuanced view. In order to distinguish between the narrow domain-specific expertise of technically brilliant performers and the innovative expertise of those working across and between domains, Hatano and Inagaki (1986) coined the term *adaptive expertise*. The example they give as an illustration is of two sushi chefs, one of whom is technically brilliant but who always produces the same food, and the other who is equally brilliant technically but who is able to produce new and innovative dishes on a regular basis. One of the aspects of this that is of interest to those working in this area is how an expert can break the mould, even if this is socially and culturally hard to do. Adaptive expertise has been termed a 'virtuoso' attribute (Schwartz *et al.* 2005). The Oxford Pocket Thesaurus gives the following synonyms for virtuosity: *brilliance, craft, éclat, expertise, finish, flair, mastery, panache, polish, skill*[4]. This list implies a combination of technical skill and charismatic attributes, along with a control of the situation implied by mastery. Those demonstrating this kind of expertise are able to be flexible and insightful, particularly in complex and dynamic situations. Adaptive experts are effective in novel situations (Holyoak 1991) and they are willing and able to transcend formal rules

---

[4] http://dictionary.reverso.net/English-synonyms (accessed June, 2010)

and procedures where the situation demands it. To this extent, the adaptive expert equates to the expert level in the model of Dreyfus and Dreyfus (1980). This flexibility might be essential in high-risk, high-uncertainty areas of practice, such as healthcare (Feltovich *et al.* 1997).

The work of Mihaly Csikszentmihalyi (1996) is relevant at this point. He introduces the notion of 'flow'. Csikszentmihalyi is a proponent of the positive psychology movement, which marked a turn away from pathological psychological responses and towards the study of positive attributes, such as happiness and creativity. Flow is a state of full absorption in what one is doing, where there is perfect synergy between the task at hand, the expertise of the individual doing the task, and the context in which it is done. This leads to a sense that the work is fluid, easy and profoundly fulfilling: a sense of harmony. When a person is in the middle of flow activities, time stands still. It might be argued that the adaptive expert is most adept at exhibiting flow, in a range of situations. To those observing, adaptive experts demonstrate a fluency of response and of engagement that marks a virtuoso performance in a range of settings.

It is important to note that this kind of expertise is not necessarily a morally or ethically 'good' phenomenon. An assassin can exhibit virtuosity and flow, as can a money launderer or a bank robber. The terms are neutral in this regard. It is the operation of them that renders the particular expert of value to society, or not.

In parallel with the theories developed above, researchers working on cognition have been trying to understand what neurological processes are employed by those who are observed to demonstrate expertise. This work has evolved from a simple linear model, somewhat as described in the early studies of Ericsson and colleagues, into a more subtle understanding. In the first instance, Chase and Simon (1973) built on so-called 'chunking theory' to demonstrate, again in chess players, that experts 'chunk' together phenomena in their area of expertise (in this case, distributions of chess pieces) so that they can quickly be moved to the short-term memory and accessed in future games. In this way, basic patterns that might be applicable in future situations are more accessible to experts, who have extended experience, and who have paid enough attention to that experience to log it cognitively. In an adaptation of this approach, Gobet and his colleague Clarkson built on earlier template theory to propose that expert chess players might both chunk data and adapt these chunks in order to test them against novel situations for an explanatory template, using schematic knowledge, and allowing them to evolve into more complex interpretive structures that explain the new situation (Gobet 1998, Gobet & Clarkson 2004).

Techniques for developing skills and knowledge in learners have been explored by a number of authors, in a range of academic domains. These include transfer, social learning, situated learning and information pick-up theory. It is beyond the scope of this chapter to discuss these in detail. However, the work of one author, Donald Schön (1983), might be directly relevant to expertise, as it is explicitly rooted in feedback and self-improvement, and recognition of the dynamic interconnectivity of the systems in which individuals live and operate. Schön has been widely cited in the healthcare literature. His seminal work, *The Reflective Practitioner*, was actually based on an observation of experts in the areas of architectural design, town planning, management, the sciences and psychotherapy.

One of the important concepts in Schöns work, 'repertoire', might be seen to be the sociological equivalent of the cognitive concept of memory chunks and templates:

> *When a practitioner makes sense of a situation he perceives to be unique, he sees it as something already present in his repertoire. . .[as an] unfamiliar, unique situation ... both similar to and different from the familiar one, without at first being able to say similar or different with respect to what. The familiar situation functions as a precedent, or a metaphor, or . . . an exemplar for the unfamiliar one.*
>
> (Schön 1983, p.138)

Despite this similarity with the insights of cognitive psychologists working in this area, there are critics of Schön, not least those who argue that the theories he proposes have not been convincingly tested in practice. However, as a metaphor for the way experts seem to think, repertoire, built up by reflection in and on action, seems to be a useful shorthand to understanding general expertise. As Schön says:'through the unintended effects of action the situation talks back . . .' (Schön 1996, p. 135).

To summarise, expert practice appears to develop over time, being facilitated through situational experiences, which the learner encounters and reflects on in order to draw upon them when making decisions for the future. The next section of this chapter examines expertise in the context of nursing, medicine and midwifery.

Expertise in the context of healthcare

Nursing expertise

Jasper (1994) has noted that 'it is apparent that when used in nursing [expertise] refers to a multitude of attributes and lacks clear definition' (p.789). In contrast to this, the work of Patricia Benner (1984), who adapted the Dreyfus and Dreyfus (1980) model of skill acquisition, offers an influential taxonomy of expertise in the field of nursing expertise.

The basis of Benner's work was a study carried out in the early 1980s, which involved interviews with nurses at different stages of practice, from novice to expert (Benner 1984). The findings of this study validated the Dreyfus and Dreyfus model in the context of nursing practice. According to Benner (2001), at novice level practitioners 'do not have any experience of the situations in which they are expected to perform' (p.20), and therefore rely on rules to guide decisions or performance. Benner refers to nursing students as novices as they 'have little understanding of the contextual meaning of the recently learned textbook terms' (p.21).

The advanced beginner has experienced enough encounters or experiences to be able to recognise important aspects of the situation and recurrent patterns. However, Benner suggests that advanced beginners are unable to identify or perform clinical tasks in order of priority: 'their nursing care needs to be backed up by nurses who have reached at least the competent level . . ., to ensure that important patient needs do not go unattended because the advanced beginner cannot yet sort out what is most important' (p. 25).

Benner suggests that practitioners become competent usually after 2–3 years, if they encounter the same or similar experiences. The competent nurse identifies long-term goals or plans for the client using analytical skills to assess the clinical situation. Benner suggests that the increasing organisation of nursing care is evident in competent practitioners: 'the conscious, deliberate planning that is characteristic of this skill level helps achieve efficiency and organisation' (p. 27).

Proficient nurses see the situation as a whole rather than in parts. Proficiency is achieved through continued clinical experience, usually over 3–5 years (Benner 2001). Proficient nurses learn from these experiences and modify plans to meet individual situations. Benner suggests that decision making becomes more refined: 'the proficient performer considers fewer options and hones in on an accurate region of the problem' (p. 29).

Finally, at the expert level the expert performer does not rely on analytical rules to guide decision making. Benner suggests that experts make accurate immediate judgements based on extensive knowledge, experience and intuition. It is this immediacy of decision making which distinguishes the expert from other levels of skill acquisition. The time taken to reach this level would appear to validate the 'rule of ten' law discussed above.

In contrast to the strict domain limits of Ericsson's model, Benner proposes that expert nurse practitioners operate in a range of roles, including the helping role, the teaching or coaching function, the diagnostic and monitoring function, effective management of rapidly changing situations, administration of monitoring therapeutic interventions and regimes, monitoring and ensuring the quality of healthcare practices, and organisation of work-role competencies (Benner 2001). The helping role includes providing emotional support, creating a climate committed to healing, encouraging and maximising patients' participation in their care, providing comfort through presence, touch and communication. The teaching-coaching function is based on the ability to assist patients to understand, cope with, accept and regain control over their illness. The diagnostic and monitoring function is facilitated through the ability to anticipate, understand and detect problems. Effective management of rapidly changing situations includes skilled performance in extreme life-threatening emergencies, being able to 'manage as well as prevent crisis' (Benner 2001, p. 119). Monitoring and ensuring the quality of healthcare practices is essential to ensure that safety standards are met, while patient needs are also met. This requires effective communication between nurses and medical personnel. The final competency relates to organisation and work role and is facilitated through co-ordination, teamwork and meeting patients' needs. This wide-ranging sphere of practice suggests that the more nuanced model of adaptive expertise is operating in the nursing context, although Benner does not use this term in her work.

While the helping role does encompass some interpersonal and caring aspects, including the important concept of 'presencing', the other six aspects are largely instrumental rather than relational. In contrast, concepts of caring have featured in the publications of Benner and her colleagues (Benner *et al.* 1996).

To summarise, Benner proposes that the transition from novice to expert is evident as practitioners become less reliant upon rules and analytical thinking to inform decision making, and instead use their wealth of clinical experience, knowledge and intuition to guide their choices. Competency or expertise has been identified in domains of practice, as described above.

Critics of this model argue that it is impossible to identify which stage nurses belong to in the expertise taxonomy or even if, indeed, they can be clearly separated into such defined broad terms (English 1993; Farrington, 1993; Edwards 1998). Specifically, Ericsson and Smith (1991a) have argued that the number of years assigned to the stages does not correlate with expertise in empirical and observational studies – some experts reach that level more quickly than the theory suggests, and others take longer (Ericsson & Smith 1991b).

Apart from discussions on the chronological development of expertise, there have been many attempts to define expertise and expert practice in various nursing disciplines (Jasper 1994; Paul & Heaslip 1995; Edwards 1998; Christensen & Hewitt-Taylor 2006a,b; Ericsson *et al.* 2007). Nelson and McGillion (2004) have argued that the use of narrative interviews and think-aloud techniques that underpin research into nursing expertise reifies nursing performance as nursing expertise.

This raises epistemological questions about how expertise is understood. Theorists have explored the relevance of Schön's work to nursing expertise, both in the field of learning and in the rejection of technical rationality as the sole base for skilful nursing practice (Kinsella 2007). More recently, Gobet and Chassy (2008) have challenged Benner's theory of expert intuition. They accept that the five-stage model offers a starting point, especially in the integration of emotion and relationality into the expertise model, but, in particular, they dispute the cognitive reality of the intuition element. Building on the chunking/template theory described above, they demonstrate how using intuition can be explained neurologically as a process of identifying patterns of health states (chunking) and then slotting them into templates. Gobet and Chassy examine the efficacy of their model against the five key template characteristics of experts: *rapid perception; lack of awareness of the process engaged; holistic understanding of the situation; experts' intuitions are normally correct; and intuition is coloured by emotions.* Template theory contextualises the chunking pattern recognition. For example, a particular event on a general medical ward, such as a fall of a male elderly patient with diabetes, might be remembered as a chunk, but when it is applied to a female patient with epilepsy, the chunk is contextualised by a different set of information. The attention of the expert is to slightly different elements of the situation in each case, as different sets of salient information are accessed from the overall chunks in the memory. Templates also allow for a phenomenon which Benner terms 'future think', where the expert rapidly assesses the likely outcomes of a range of possible actions (using different templates), before taking the chosen course in each specific case.

As the overview in this section suggests, until recently, much of the research into nursing expertise has taken a phenomenological standpoint. In contrast, researchers looking into medical expertise have started from a cognitive perspective. The next section examines this body of work.

Medical expertise

In a comprehensive overview of medical judgement and competence, Eraut and du Boulay (2001) provide an account of a range of theories of expertise relating to medical practice. They propose a model in which knowledge, competence and judgement are key components. They conclude that:

> *Key features of expertise include the importance of case-based experience, the rapid retrieval of information from memory attributable to its superior organisation, the development of standard patterns of reasoning and*

problem-solving, quick recognition of which approach to use and when, awareness of bias and fallibility; and the ability to track down, evaluate and use evidence from research and case-specific data ... (section 0.2(1))

This interpretation of expertise is rooted in a psychological and neurological model. As an example, while 'communication skills' are included under the theme of 'competency', issues of relationship and reciprocity are not mentioned.

Despite this apparently instrumental take on medical expertise, Eruat and du Boulay do recognise from the papers in their review that doctors do not function in predictable, certain environments, in which practice can always be based on predetermined guidelines or protocols. A number of the authors cited in their review postulate that medical experts adopt the use of so-called 'illness scripts' (Schmidt *et al.* 1990; Custers *et al.* 1996; Schmidt & Rikers 2007). This theory was developed using models of reasoning based on cognitive psychology. It pays attention to goal-directed knowledge structures, that emerge from prior experiences:

> ... *illness scripts' [are] decisions for individuals ... based on the use of chunks or pictures of past experiences in future clinical reasoning, as opposed to the use of linear evidence based medicine.*
>
> (Custers et al. 1996)

In their original paper on illness scripts, Schmidt and colleagues propose that this way of reasoning is not concerned with causes and symptoms, but with 'a wealth of clinically relevant information about disease, its consequences, and the context under which illness develops' (Schmidt *et al.* 1990, p.611). In passing, this has an interesting resonance with recent concepts of realist research (what works, for whom, in what context; Pawson *et al.* 2005). The rapid acceptance of realist research and narrative medicine theories (Greenhalgh & Hurwitz 1998) might be explained by the fact that these non-linear approaches make sense in terms of script theory, and that script theory does indeed explain how expert doctors think.

Indeed, the original construct of script theory, proposed by Silvan Tomkins (1987), depends strongly on the impact of the emotional affect of a scene or event as a marking mechanism that enables that event to be stored as a script. Narrative is a device that strongly links emotional affect with events and memory. Following up this lead, Charlin *et al.* 2000, 2007 describe the illness scripts as a special case of script theory, but they pay minimal attention to the affective elements of the theory.

Schmidt and Rikers (2007) reviewed 30 years of research into the acquisition of medical knowledge. They conclude that biomedical knowledge becomes encapsulated through experience, and then integrated into illness scripts. More recently, this team has developed a tool based on the instrumental elements of script theory, to compare the judgement of trainees against that of expert neurologists, based on complex clinical scenarios (Lubarsky *et al.* 2009). They found that less experienced practitioners did not score as well as more experienced ones, and that the tool discriminated between different levels of seniority. It is not clear if adding an affective element to the tool would increase its discriminatory capacity.

Illness script theory has obvious links to the chunking theory discussed above. In a different take on the general chunking/template/patterns of reasoning theory, Kushniruk and colleagues (1998) have proposed the so-called 'small worlds' hypothesis. In this theory, small worlds are subsets of disease categories, and the features that distinguish them. The argument is that experts make limited comparisons between the small worlds they know and clinical cases that present to them. In the study undertaken by Kushniruk *et al.*, experts rapidly selected 'small worlds' of plausible diagnostic hypotheses in each case that was presented to them. They discriminated among these alternatives stepwise and efficiently. Non-experts tended to select a wider range of possible hypotheses, and to be less discriminating in choosing between them.

More recently, Mamede and colleagues (2008) have discussed the role of reflection in practice in relation to medical diagnosis, and the development of expertise. In their study of 42 internal medicine residents in hospitals in two states in the north east of Brazil, participants were asked to diagnose clinical cases based on either pattern recognition or reflective reasoning. They found that, although reflective practice did not always differentiate effective diagnosis, in cases of complex and unusual cases there was a clear positive effect of this way of reasoning. This work suggests that medical expertise (and, possibly, healthcare expertise in general) is a mix of instrumental, pattern-based and context-specific reasoning, linked in complex cases with reflective, affect-sensitive approaches. The next section examines the case of midwifery expertise, taking these findings into account.

Maternity care expertise

Although midwifery may have similarities with both nursing and medical practice, the scope and sphere of midwifery are different from either of these. There is less empirical evidence on midwifery expertise than for either medicine or nursing. In the light of this, a meta-synthesis of the literature in this area has recently been undertaken (Downe *et al.* 2007). The aim of the review was to synthesise completed

English-language studies published between 1970 and 2005, relating to constructs of maternity care in the context of practitioners who are practising 'beyond the ordinary'. Databases, journal publications and national research resources were searched by hand, or electronically, using defined search terms, and inclusion and exclusion criteria.

The findings identified that the terms 'expert', 'exemplary' and 'experienced' were used interchangeably by some authors in this field. Seven good-quality papers were included. Ten themes were eventually identified by consensus. Three intersecting concepts were identified from these themes: wisdom, skilled practice and enacted vocation. The three overarching themes were not context specific. They transcended locations of work, such as the labour ward or home birth, and philosophies such as 'a midwife is a midwife is a midwife' or 'midwives are (only) the experts in the normal'.

Discussion

Theorists and researchers have been fascinated with the concept of expertise for many years. The main schools of thought seem to fall into two camps. On the one hand, cognitive researchers working largely from an epistemological position of positivism have examined the effect of repeated practice, and of methods of organising and retrieving memory on expertise. On the other hand, phenomenologists working from an interpretivist stance have sought to describe the nature of expertise as it is manifest in actual practice. There seems to be general agreement that experts learn effectively from past experience, and that they have rapid access to that experience in some form, such as chunking or cognitive scripts. Experts also seem to have the capacity to fit historical patterns of experience into possible templates for current and future action in a more efficient way than non-experts.

However, this does not explain the difference between those who are expert in one specific domain and those experts who seem to be able to transcend domains of practice. The theory of adaptive expertise goes some way towards explaining the difference between technical experts, who may be novices in all areas but the one in which they are practised and efficient, and those who can translate their expertise between at least some domains. It is possible that this explains the difference between an expert surgeon, for example, and an expert general practitioner. In the former case, the expertise is technical and instrumental. In the latter, it is nuanced and general, and more likely to be influenced by affective components, such as the relationship with the patient.

The components identified in the meta-synthesis of midwifery expertise referred to in this chapter may be useful in describing elements of expertise that are likely to cross domains, and to be strongly expressed in adaptive experts in healthcare. In this specific case of midwifery, where normal childbirth is a primary concern, it can be hypothesised that 'wellness scripts' might be operating, particularly for those who regularly cross boundaries between biomedically and sociologically orientated practice – those termed postmodern midwives by Davis-Floyd (Davis-Floyd & Davis 1997). This is addressed in more detail in the next chapter. Midwifery, nursing and general practice also offer a locus for reintroducing the emotional component of pattern retrieval, in a return to the affective theory that underpins script theory. As a starting point for examining the utility of realist research and narrative-based medicine, this theory might be a useful basis for research into effective practice in the future. It also may explain the basis of expertise that has been expressed as 'skilled help from the heart' (El-Nemer *et al.* 2006).

Conclusion

This chapter has examined some of the key theories in the development of expertise. The next chapter summarises an empirical research study that was designed to establish the nature of midwifery expertise, building on the meta-synthesis by Downe and colleagues (2007). The findings of the study are contextualised by the theories of expertise that have been identified in this chapter, with the aim of developing a more useful understanding of midwifery expertise for the future.

References

Benner P (1984) *From Novice to Expert. Excellence and Power in Clinical Nursing Practice.* New Jersey, Prentice-Hall.

Benner P (2001) *From Novice to Expert. Excellence and Power in Clinical Nursing Practice.* Commemorative edition. New Jersey, Prentice-Hall.

Benner P, Tanner CA, Chesla CA (1996) *Expertise in Nursing Practice – Caring, Clinical Judgement, and Ethics.* New York, Springer.

Bloom BS (1985). *Developing Talent in Young People.* New York, Ballantine.

Charlin B, Tardif J, Boshuizen HP (2000) Scripts and medical diagnostic knowledge: theory and applications for clinical reasoning instruction and research. *Academic Medicine* 75(2): 182–90.

Charlin B, Boshuizen HP, Custers EJ, Feltovich PJ (2007) Scripts and clinical reasoning. *Medical Education* 41(12): 1178–84.

Chase WG, Simon HA (1973) The mind's eye in chess. In Chase WB (ed) *Visual Information Processing.* New York, Academic Press, 215–81.

Christensen M, Hewitt-Taylor J (2006a) Defining the expert ICU nurse. *Intensive and Critical Care Nursing* 22: 301–7.

Christensen M, Hewitt-Taylor J (2006b) From expert to tasks, expert nursing practice redefined? Issues in clinical nursing. *Journal of Clinical Nursing* 15(12): 1531–9.

Csikszentmihalyi M (1996) *Creativity: Flow and the Psychology of Discovery and Invention*. New York, Harper Perennial.

Custers EJ, Boshuizen HP, Schmidt HG (1996) The influence of medical expertise, case typicality, and illness script component on case processing and disease probability estimates. *Memory and Cognition* 24: 384–99.

Davis-Floyd R, Davis E (1997) Intuition as authoritative knowledge in midwifery and home birth. In Davis-Floyd R, Sargent C (eds) *Childbirth and Authoritative Knowledge: Cross-Cultural Perspectives*. Berkeley, CA, University of California Press, 315–49.

Downe S, Simpson L, Trafford K (2007) Expert intrapartum care: a meta-synthesis. *Journal of Advanced Nursing* 57(2): 127–40.

Dreyfus HL, Dreyfus SE (1986) *Mind Over Machine. The Power of Human Intuition and Expertise in the Era of the Computer*. Oxford, Blackwell.

Dreyfus SE, Dreyfus HL (1980) *A Five-Stage Model of the Mental Activities Involved in Directed Skill Acquisition*. www.stormingmedia.us/15/1554/A155480.html (accessed June, 2010).

Edwards SD (1998) *Philosophical Issues in Nursing*. London, Macmillan.

El-Nemer A, Downe S, Small N (2006) She would help me from the heart: an ethnography of Egyptian women in labour. *Social Science and Medicine* 62(1): 81–92.

English I (1993) Intuition as a function of the expert nurse: a critique of Benner's novice to expert model. *Journal of Advanced Nursing* 18(3): 387–93.

Eraut M, du Boulay B (2001) *Developing the Attributes of Medical Professional Judgement and Competence*. Report to the Department of Health. www.informatics.sussex.ac.uk/users/bend/doh/reporthtml.html (accessed June, 2010).

Ericsson KA (1996) The acquisition of expert performance: an introduction to some of the issues. In Ericsson KA (ed) *The Road to Excellence: The Acquisition of Expert Performance in the Arts and Sciences, Sports, and Games*. London, Psychology Press, 1–50.

Ericsson KA, Smith J (eds) (1991a) *Toward a General Theory of Expertise: Prospects and Limits*. Cambridge, Cambridge University Press.

Ericsson KA, Smith J (1991b) Prospects and limits of the empirical study of expertise: an introduction. In Ericsson KA, Smith J (eds) *Toward a General Theory of Expertise: Prospects and Limits*. Cambridge, Cambridge University Press, 1–38.

Ericsson KA, Krampe R, Tesch-Römer C (1993) The role of deliberate practice in the acquisition of expert performance. *Psychological Review* 100: 363–406.

Ericsson KA, Whyte J, Ward P (2007) Expert performance in nursing: reviewing research on expertise in nursing within the framework of the expert-performance approach. *Advances in Nursing Science* 30(1): e58–e71.

Farrington A (1993) Intuition and expert clinical practice in nursing. *British Journal of Nursing* 2(4): 228–33.

Feltovich PJ, Spiro RJ, Coulson RL (1997) Issues of expert flexibility in contexts characterized by complexity and change. In Feltovich PJ, Ford KM, Hoffman RR (eds) *Expertise in Context*. Menlo Park, CA, AAAI Press/MIT Press, 126–46.

Gobet F (1998) Expert memory: a comparison of four theories. *Cognition* 66(2): 115–52.

Gobet F, Chassy P (2008) Towards an alternative to Benner's theory of expert intuition in nursing: a discussion paper. *International Journal of Nursing Studies* 45(1): 129–39.

Gobet F, Clarkson G (2004) Chunks in expert memory: evidence for the magical number four ... or is it two? *Memory* 12(6): 732–47.

Greenhalgh T, Hurwitz B (1998) *Narrative Based Medicine*. London, BMJ Books.

Hardy S, Garbett R, Titchen A, Manley K (2002) Exploring nursing expertise: nurses talk nursing. *Nursing Inquiry* 9(3): 196–202.

Hatano G, Inagaki K (1986) Two courses of expertise. *Child Development And Education in Japan* 262–72.

Holyoak KJ (1991) Symbolic connectionism: toward third-generation theories of expertise. In Ericsson KA, Smith J (eds) *Toward a General Theory of Expertise: Prospects and Limits*. Cambridge, Cambridge University Press, 301–35.

Howe MJA (1999) *Genius Explained*. Cambridge, Cambridge University Press.

Jasper M (1994) Expert: a discussion of the implications of the concept as used in nursing. *Journal of Advanced Nursing* 20: 769–76.

Kinsella EA (2007) Technical rationality in Schön's reflective practice: dichotomous or non-dualistic epistemological position. *Nursing Philosophy* 8(2): 102–13.

Kushniruk AW, Patel VL, Marley AA (1998) Small worlds and medical expertise: implications for medical cognition and knowledge engineering. *International Journal of Medical Informatics* 49(3): 255–71.

Lubarsky S, Chalk C, Kazitani D, Gagnon R, Charlin B (2009) The Script Concordance Test: a new tool assessing clinical judgement in neurology. *Canadian Journal of Neurological Science* 36(3): 326–31.

Mamede S, Schmidt HG, Penaforte JC (2008) Effects of reflective practice on the accuracy of medical diagnoses. *Medical Education* 42(5): 468–75.

Nelson S, McGillion M (2004) Expertise or performance? Questioning the rhetoric of contemporary narrative use in nursing. *Journal of Advanced Nursing* 47(6): 631–8.

Paul R, Heaslip P (1995) Critical thinking and intuitive nursing practice. *Journal of Advanced Nursing* 33: 40–7.

Pawson R, Greenhalgh T, Harvey G, Walshe K (2005) Realist review – a new method of systematic review designed for complex policy interventions. *Journal of Health Services Research and Policy* 10(suppl 1): 21–34.

Peden-McAlpine C (1999) Expert thinking in nursing practice: implications for supporting expertise. *Nursing and Health Sciences* 1: 131–7.

Schmidt HG, Rikers RM (2007) How expertise develops in medicine: knowledge encapsulation and illness script formation. *Medical Education* 41(12): 1133–9.

Schmidt HG, Norman GR, Boshuizen HP (1990) A cognitive perspective on medical expertise: theory and implication. *Academic Medicine* 65(10): 611–21.

Schön D (1983) *The Reflective Practitioner. How Professionals Think in Action.* London, Temple Smith.

Schön D (1996) *Educating the Reflective Practitioner: Toward a New Design for Teaching and Learning in the Professions.* San Francisco, Jossey-Bass.

Schwartz DL, Bransford JD, Sears D (2005) Efficiency and innovation in transfer. In Mestre J (ed) *Transfer of Learning from a Modern Multidisciplinary Perspective.* Greenwich, CT, Information Age Publishing, 1–51.

Simon HA, Chase WG (1973) Skill in chess. *American Scientist* 61: 394–403.

Tomkins S (1987) Script theory. In Arnoff J, Rabin AI, Zucker RA (eds) *The Emergence of Personality.* New York, Springer, 147–216.

Chapter 6
Expertise in Intrapartum Midwifery Practice

Louise Simpson and Soo Downe

Introduction

As Chapter 5 has indicated, there is a wide range of theories and scholarly texts that address the nature of expertise in general. Some of this has been applied in a healthcare context. There is some research evidence relating to the nature of midwifery expertise, and this has recently been subject of a meta-synthesis, as described previously (Downe *et al.* 2007). However, although the international definition of the midwife is widely cited (ICM 2005), debate remains as to how this should be applied in practice. In the UK, this debate was sharpened by proposals for advanced level practice in the 1990s (Macleod Clark *et al.* 2009) and, more recently, by discussion about the role of the consultant midwife (Coster *et al.* 2006; Humphreys *et al.* 2007). To date, higher-level recordable qualifications in midwifery have been rejected by the profession, although midwives are employed in specialist roles and consultant posts.

This chapter is based on the findings of a study of midwives' views of expert midwifery practice, and of the related meta-synthesis that was introduced in Chapter 5.

Aims, methods and emerging themes

The aim of the study was to explore the nature of intrapartum midwifery expertise, in order to illuminate the essential characteristics and skills

Essential Midwifery Practice: Leadership, Expertise and Collaborative Working,
first edition. Edited by Soo Downe, Sheena Byrom and Louise Simpson
Published 2011 by Blackwell Publishing Ltd.
© 2011 Blackwell Publishing Ltd.

that facilitate optimal birth outcomes for women. An interpretive phenomenological approach was used. Both group and individual interviews were held. Twenty four practising midwives (E–H grades[1]), located in the north west of England, employed within two midwifery-led units and two consultant units, provided the sampling frame for this research. In order to capture a wide range of experiences and meanings, one consultant-led unit had a higher than UK national average rate of normal birth (site A) (as defined by Birth Choice UK[2]), while the other had a lower than UK average rate of normal birth (site B). Both midwifery-led units were free-standing[3] midwifery-led units (sites C and D). The rationale for the inclusion of both midwifery-led and consultant units was that they covered a range of philosophical approaches to childbirth, as demonstrated by either much higher than average or much lower than average rates of normal birth.

The group interview guide consisted of three research areas that were to be addressed: midwifery expertise in general, normal birth and expertise in normality. Under each section, prompts were listed to guide the discussion if required. The interview guide acted as a standard starting point for all four group interviews. The guide used during the individual interviews consisted of one open-ended question: 'I want you to think of someone who you regard an expert in intrapartum care. Tell me about your encounters with that person (or a specific encounter that best demonstrates his/her expertise'. This facilitated the participants' spontaneous accounts of their experience of or encounter with expert practice. Two further questions were added to explore expertise in high-risk and low-risk environments.

Four themes emerged from the findings: wisdom, skilled practice, enacted vocation and connected companionship. Further analysis suggested that there were three domains of expert midwifery practice, based on the accounts of the respondents: physiological expertise, technical expertise and integrated expertise. Integrated expertise appears to be the strongest of the three, being characterised by the experts' ability to work across boundaries of normality, and through differing models of care, in order to promote optimal birth outcomes for women.

The rest of this chapter examines the findings in depth, as a basis for developing a theory of midwifery expertise for the future.

[1] Prior to the implementation of a new grading system in 2006 (Agenda for Change), practising midwives were graded from E to H grade, with E-grade midwives regarded as more junior and H grade usually managers. However, the grades were not necessarily determined by years of experience. Midwives ascended through the grades via promotion.

[2] Birth Choice UK. www.birthchoiceuk.com (accessed June, 2010).

[3] Free-standing midwifery-led units are run by midwives and provide care for low-risk women. There are no obstetricians available on site. Women requiring obstetric intervention would require transfer to the nearest consultant unit.

The nature of midwifery expertise

Wisdom

The overarching theme of wisdom incorporated knowledge, education, experience and personal attributes. These are addressed in detail later in this section.

Although the concept of wisdom has been explored by various researchers (Tritten 1992; Lauder 1994; Litchfield 1999), an agreed definition does not yet exist (Ardelt 2004). Ardelt (2004) proposes a three-dimensional personality characteristic of wisdom (cognitive, reflective and affective):

> *The cognitive dimension of wisdom refers to the desire to know the truth and attain a deeper understanding of life ... the reflective component of wisdom represents self-examination, self-awareness, self-insight and the ability to look at the phenomena and events from different perspectives ... and finally the affective component consists of a person's sympathetic and compassionate love for others.*
>
> (Ardelt 2004, p.275)

The desire to gain knowledge, the ability to learn from experience, and the ability to be motivated to seek new knowledge and experiences appear to fit within the cognitive dimension of wisdom. The ability to be reflective and reflexive in order to give individualised care to meet the individual needs of the woman and her family appears to fit within the reflective dimension. Finally, the ability to make connected relationships with women and colleagues, founded on trust, honesty and mutual respect, appears to fit the affective component.

The following quote from the study appears to represent what is meant by the concept of 'wisdom'.

> *... And you learn a bit from each colleague ... You sort of take a bit from each one, don't you ... You know, I always think I learnt from (mentions midwife's name) ... she's a very gentle, laid-back sort of person, who's retired now ... being with her and somebody who was in the second stage of labour, and you'd think she was on a walk outside in the countryside on a sunny day, sort of thing. And I sat on a stool for the first time in the labour ward and we just chatted ... with the lady... I just learnt to be relaxed and not interfere, whereas prior to that it would be like the legs on our hips and give a good push ... and she just undid that 18 months, which was really good.*
>
> (Group interview, midwifery-led unit D)

This echoes the reflective and affective components of wisdom. Personal attributes such as 'gentle' and 'laid-back' describe the characteristics of the expert. She facilitates a calm, relaxed environment, and establishes relationships with women through effective communication. The participant suggests that the experience of working with this expert changed and influenced her way of practising. The phrase 'and she just undid that 18 months' is a powerful statement, as it suggests that midwives' routine practices can be challenged and changed by observing expert practice.

Knowledge and experience

Eraut (1994) identified two facets of knowledge: 'knowing that' and 'knowing how'. 'Knowing that' refers to a fundamental knowledge base or theory, and 'knowing how' refers to being able to do the job. Eraut suggests that professional knowledge integrates the two and, together with a unique understanding of the individual patient, determines expertise (Downe *et al.* 2007).

Ardelt (2004) argues that:

> . . . *intellectual or theoretical knowledge is knowledge that is understood only at the intellectual level, whereas wisdom is understood at the experiential level. It is only when the individual realises (i.e. experiences) the truth of this preserved knowledge that the knowledge is re-transformed into wisdom and makes the person wise(r).*
>
> (p.260)

Findings from the study suggested that expert midwives possess a sound knowledge base that is continuously being updated through ongoing education and research. Emphasis was placed on the importance of updating knowledge in order to stimulate mental ability. It appears to be the motivation or desire to learn that differentiates the expert from the non-expert. Kennedy (2000) revealed similar findings in her study, where 'experts' demonstrated 'intellectual curiosity', as they continuously searched for educational opportunities.

However, expertise appears to derive from something more than possessing knowledge or having experience. Kennedy (1987) argues that although expertise evolves and develops with experience, 'expertise cannot be assumed to develop automatically through years of service' (p.175). This concept was supported by the study respondents:

> *I think . . . no offence to some of the newly qualified midwives, no they are not experts, no they are not experts as they have not got the quality of experience. That comes and it comes sooner or later, doesn't it . . . you don't have to have 20 years to be an expert . . .*
>
> (Group interview, midwifery-led unit C)

> *And equally we've had midwives who've been in this unit 25 years who you wouldn't consider experts. . .*
>
> (Group interview, consultant unit A)

The development of expertise seems to depend on the quality of experience and not on time-serving. In this context, quality refers to the diversity of the experience and how this is internalized. Ang (2002) supports this claim by proposing that 'the progression from novice to expert nurse depends on the ability to learn from experience and to apply the knowledge when faced with a similar situation' (p.493). Benner (2001) suggests that experiences require 'processing' in order to have an impact on future practice or behaviour. Thus, expertise derives from the practitioner's ability to examine and analyse performance, with the objective of refining practice (Benner 2001). In order for this to occur, experts demonstrate the ability to be both reflective and reflexive in their practice.

Education

Eraut (1994) suggests that expertise derives from both experience and formal education. The meta-synthesis of studies of midwifery expertise that preceded this study (Downe *et al.* 2007) found very little evidence of the importance of formal education to the development of expertise. Although there is literature debating the significance of route of entry to nursing and midwifery (pre-registration or postregistration) with regard to confidence or competency (Alexander 1993; Fleming & Milde 2000), this aspect did not appear in the papers located by the search strategy or in the qualitative study.

It is possible that education is being taken for granted as a core requirement on which expertise would be built. Although the 'degree' itself was suggested to facilitate further learning and development, participants expressed the view that possessing the qualification of a midwifery degree was not a predetermining factor to the development of expertise. It may be argued that experts exist in the absence of academic qualifications. This appears to challenge the current culture of 'super-valuing' higher education. The key factor appeared to be the ability to reflect on and integrate knowledge acquired through education and experience, rather than a formal qualification *per se*.

Personal attributes

Barwise (1998) suggests that personality type cannot be ignored, as each midwife has unique perceptions and experiences. The following personal attributes, qualities or characteristics were proposed by participants to be characteristic of expert practice: calm and confident; advocate; approachable; gentle; caring; good communicator; compassionate; kind; committed; enthusiastic; forward thinking; motivated;

dynamic; friend; adaptable; flexible; supportive. The most commonly described characteristic was the ability to be kind or caring to women and colleagues.

Experts were frequently described as being calm and relaxed in their approach. In an apparent paradox, as well as being calm, experts were suggested to be dynamic and motivated, often doing things beyond their call of duty. Experts were suggested to be dedicated or even devoted to midwifery.

These attributes resonate with the concept of vocation. Arguably, the vocational ideal in healthcare has been marginalised by advancing technology and social and cultural change, and displaced by professional projects (Salvage 2004; Wright 2004). Despite the shifting context of midwifery care, these results suggest that, as midwives move through being a novice to becoming an expert, they may revalue the art of vocation.

Summary of findings relating to wisdom

This section has explored how knowledge, education, experience and the personal characteristics or attributes of the midwife are integrated to produce wisdom. Experts appear to be highly motivated and dynamic, constantly acquiring new knowledge and skills. This aspect of expertise appears to fit within the cognitive dimension of wisdom as proposed by Ardelt (2004). The ability to reflect on and learn from experiences is consistent with the reflective aspect of wisdom, and denotes expert practice. Finally, the affective component of wisdom is demonstrated through valuing the 'art' of midwifery, where emphasis is placed on caring and nurturing.

Skilled practice

As Shallow (2001) notes, 'Expertise is not simply about performing a particular procedure or set of procedures quickly or efficiently' (p.237). Dreyfus (2004) argues that it is the ability to make refined, subtle decisions that discriminates the expert from the proficient performer. Experts demonstrate the ability to 'grasp the situation directly, recognize salient aspects, and ignore irrelevant ones' (Shapiro 1998, p.13).

Findings from this study have identified four codes that captured the meaning of 'skilled practice': technical and fundamental midwifery skills; confidence; competence; and judgement and decision-making skills. Although some of these appear to be interlinked, each will be explored separately in this section.

Technical and fundamental midwifery skills

Henderson (1969) described the truly excellent practitioner as 'one who has mastered the many technical skills and who uses her emotional and technical responses in a unique design that suits the particular needs of the person she serves' (p.76). Experts in this study were observed to possess both technical skills and the more subtle skills of keeping birth normal. Both technical and fundamental midwifery skills were valued, transcending across the boundaries of normal and pathological. Although it may be argued that midwifery skills may be regarded by society as inferior to technological knowledge (Woodward 1997), these subtle midwifery skills in fact appear to be fundamental in terms of facilitating positive birth outcomes, and in the development of expert practice.

Confidence

The participants reported that expert midwives were confident practitioners. Experts were reported to demonstrate adaptability in their ability to work in any setting, confidence in making decisions, and in their ability to 'act' or 'not to act':

> *I read somewhere that the definition of a good midwife is somebody who has good hands and knows when to sit on them* (laughter). *Well, yeah. But equally knows when to use them.*
>
> (Group interview, midwifery-led unit D)

This confidence of 'acting' or 'not acting' was identified in the literature review. Kennedy (2002) has referred to not acting as 'the art of doing nothing well'. In parallel with this skill, experts demonstrated confidence and competence in their ability to take charge of emergency situations.

Competence

Although there is literature examining the nature of competence in nursing and midwifery, there is controversy surrounding its definition (Worth-Butler *et al.* 1995). Newble (1992) simplifies competence as the 'mastery of the body of relevant knowledge and the acquisition of a range of relevant skills' (p.226).

Participants in this study suggested that expert midwives were able to recognise their own limitations, were able to work in any setting, and demonstrated competence in their ability to deal with the uncertainty and unpredictability of labour. We first identified this ability to deal with uncertainty in the prior literature review, and defined it as 'reflexive competence' (Downe *et al.* 2007). Reflexive competence captures the expert's ability to make rapid decisions that are not dependent on standard protocols or routine techniques. It also doesn't depend on leadership.

Although the participants suggested that experts were able to demonstrate leadership abilities, including being innovative, forward thinking, reflective, being a role model, having good communication skills, trusting others and being trusted by colleagues, they did not necessarily have to be regarded formally as a leader. Indeed, experts seemed to be particularly skilled in letting others take the lead. This included both colleagues and childbearing women.

Judgement and decision making

The very complexity of decision making, especially in the dynamic process of labour and birth, necessitates shortcuts in reasoning (Cioffi & Markham 1997). Harbison (2000) argues:

> To understand the activity of clinical decision making, one has to draw upon knowledge from such diverse disciplines as cognitive and social psychology, philosophy, artificial intelligence, and statistical theories. In doing so, one has to be willing to range across the 'art' versus 'science' divide: and to value both qualitative and quantitative paradigms.
>
> (p.132)

Thus, the key to expert performance lies in the individual's memory and perception of situations as a whole rather than in their ability to solve problems quickly or efficiently. Expert clinical judgement is based on the ability to recognise subtle likenesses to previous experiences, and relate them to the current clinical situation (Dreyfus & Dreyfus 1986).

Participants in the study suggested that expert decision making was based on a combination of knowledge, experience and intuition. Experts made decisions in situations that were often unpredictable, requiring dynamic and often rapid responses. Adaptability was seen as an essential skill when dealing with the unpredictability and dynamic process of labour. Participants observed that experts made decisions based on their own clinical judgements, rather than routinely and strictly adhering to policies or guidelines. Although they practised within boundaries of safety, and within the sphere of their practice, their practice was not determined or influenced by the fear of litigation.

This ability to be in tune with women, provide the right balance between control and support, and to make intuitive judgements requires an inner connectedness within the midwife herself, and also between the woman and the midwife. The expert is able to negotiate the balance between control and support, make judgements about whether to stand back, allowing labour to progress naturally, or to take charge and intervene when necessary.

Similar findings were reported in the meta-synthesis (Downe *et al.* 2007). Based on the prior research literature, experts made judgements during the process of the labour itself, and were observed across a spectrum of 'waiting for the woman' at one extreme and 'seizing the woman' at the other (Lundgren & Dahlberg 2002).

Paradoxically, participants in this study noted that experts sometimes used specific techniques as a way of protecting the woman against the perceived risk of further medical intervention. This is a process that has been termed 'ironic intervention' (Annendale 1998). It is not clear if women make judgements about whether the expert technique is the 'lesser of two evils'.

Summary of findings related to skilled practice

This section has explored how technical and fundamental midwifery skills, confidence, competence, and judgement and decision-making skills create the theme of 'skilled practice'. Although respondents believed that they practised within the boundaries of safety, and within their sphere of practice, their practice did not appear to be defensive due to the fear of litigation. Decisions were reflexive and reflective, were not dependent upon routine policies or protocols, and were based on a combination of knowledge, prior experiences and intuition.

Enacted vocation

The word 'vocation' comes from the Latin verb *vocare* meaning 'to call' and may be defined as a summons or strong inclination to a particular course of action (Salvage 2004). Nursing and midwifery have appeared to move away from vocational qualities such as dedication, compassion, kindness and humility, placing emphasis on science and technology instead (Allen 2004). According to White (2002), 'vocations do not require practitioners to act "above and beyond" occupational norms; they require a commitment to, and identification with, the virtues and values of the occupation' (p.283).

The term 'enacted vocation' was used in the review as it appeared that as practitioners became more expert, they appeared to '(re)value and to express qualities such as trust, belief and courage, to be more willing to act on intuitive gestalt insights, and to prioritise connected relationships over displays of technical brilliance'(Downe *et al.* 2007, p.136).

The theme of enacted vocation encompassed belief and trust in birth, courage and intuition.

Belief and trust in birth

It has been argued that trust is one of the fundamental aspects of midwifery (Kirkham 2000; Calvert 2002; Gould 2004). Trust has many interpretations and meanings. As a component of midwifery care, it may be described as 'a context from which to provide care, promote normal processes, ensure informed decision making, empower women no matter what choices they make, and, when the woman's choice and midwife's philosophy differ, as a bridge from which to provide effective midwifery care' (Thorstensen 2000).

Participants identified various aspects of trust that were inherent in experts. They suggested that expert midwives held a firm belief and trust in the normal processes of birth, and that their skills included the capacity to instil confidence in women and their partners, and to empower women to trust and believe in their own ability to give birth. It was felt that it was the role of the expert midwife to instil trust and belief in colleagues through the promotion of natural childbirth practices, promoting initiatives or practices such as home birth and midwifery-led care as a way of increasing midwives', and women's, confidence and trust in normal birth.

Courage

Clancy (2003) proposes that as one of the four cardinal virtues (prudence, justice, courage, temperance), 'courage acts as a stabilizing factor for the other three' (p.128). Courage appears to be strongly related to leadership (Heischman 2002). However, courage is not the same as foolhardiness (Mavroidis 2003). Although practitioners may appear to demonstrate courage when making decisions which involve uncertainty and risk, they must have knowledge and wisdom, and be aware of risk and the consequences of actions taken (Heischman 2002).

Courage appears to be an important aspect of expertise. Experts were reported to be courageous and dynamic in their ability to challenge protocols, cultural norms or unit philosophy, and routine practices. The participants also suggested that experts demonstrated courage in their ability to make decisions based on intuition. Similar findings were also revealed in the literature review (Downe *et al.* 2007) and, specifically, in the work of Berg & Dahlberg (2001) and James *et al.* (2003).

Intuition

There are various definitions of the term 'intuition' in the published literature (Benner & Tanner 1987; Young 1987; Rew 1990; King & Appleton 1997). It has been described by Truman (2002) as 'a specific mode of thinking that evolves from the merger of knowledge, skill and experience, and is not always supported by evidence' (p.23).

Benner (2001) argues that intuitive decision making is an important characteristic of expert practice. However, King & Appleton (1997) argue that research suggests that intuition appears to be evident in practitioners ranging from student to expert practitioner and state: 'participants pointed out that "gut feelings" are often present in students and newly qualified nurses' (p.199).

Participants in our study suggested that in order for intuition and thus expertise to develop, midwives must encounter and experience the physiological or natural processes of labour, so that they are able to recognise the normal process of labour, and when deviations from the normal occur. Thus, experts appeared to sense the situation using their hands, eyes and ears, rather than relying on monitors or machines.

Although participants were unable to explain where intuitive knowledge came from, they suggested that intuition was facilitated through prior experiences, and through the midwife–woman relationship. As in an earlier study conducted by Davis-Floyd (1996), participants in this study recognised the importance of intuition, but were apprehensive about their capacity to justify decisions made on this basis:

> It's having the background knowledge as well, because your gut feeling is whatever, but you have to be able to back that up because you know you couldn't stand up and defend yourself: 'Oh well, I just thought that'. Your gut feelings don't matter in court.
>
> (Group interview, midwifery-led unit D)

Intuition requires an inner connectedness within the midwife herself, and also between the woman and the midwife. This was also evident in Davis-Floyd's (1996) study where she claimed that: 'intuition ... emerges out of their own inner connectedness to the deepest bodily and spiritual aspects of their being, as well as out of their physical and psychic connections to the mother and child' (p.260). Baylor (1997) argues that this connectedness is an intrinsic property of intuition, and essential to the development of expertise.

Summary of findings related to enacted vocation

Participants suggested that experts use and value technical, fundamental and vocational skills in order to integrate the art and science of midwifery, and to provide effective midwifery care. Experts are highly intuitive and possess a strong belief in their own skill and ability. They trust the birth process and demonstrate courage when challenging cultural norms and routine intervention. They are skilled in using their senses to detect deviations from normal, and to facilitate a connected relationship with labouring women.

Connected companionship

The relationships formed between the expert midwife and her colleagues, those formed with women for whom she cares, and the consequent creation of an environment of mutual trust have formed the concept of 'connected companionship' (Downe *et al.* 2007). Connection refers to physical, emotional, intellectual and psychic relationships (Davis-Floyd 1996). Davis-Floyd suggests that the holistic midwife values inter- and intrapersonal connection, and that the connected relationship may be described as a dance (Davis-Floyd 1996).

Baylor (1997) suggests that the 'formulation of connection is based upon a person's knowledge structures which reflect his/her level of expertise' (p.188). The term 'companionship' is chosen as it necessitates a relationship which is founded on mutual respect and trust. The term 'connected companionship' denotes a relationship that is characterised by profound caring and deep understanding. It denotes relationships between the expert and the woman, the expert and her colleagues, and the relationship between the woman, the expert and the birth environment.

Midwife–woman relationship

Fleming (1998) stated that 'the practice of midwifery itself represents a coming together of midwife and woman' (p.139), with each relationship formed being unique. In contemporary midwifery practice, 'midwives are expected to work in partnership with women, meet women's emotional needs and facilitate women's informed choice' (Hunter 2006, p.320).

Despite the significance placed on the value of the midwife–woman relationship, there appears to be little authoritative research or scholarship in this area.

Participants in the study recognised the importance of the midwife–woman relationship, and suggested that it is built on trust and equality, and facilitated through continuity of carer. The terms 'partnership' and 'friendship' were commonly used to describe the relationship. These terms have also been cited in the literature (Walsh 1999; Pairman 2000). 'Friendship', is used to describe a relationship based on 'reciprocal love and intimacy, trust, warmth and genuine concern' (Pairman 2000, p.224). A friendship is usually a relationship which is voluntarily entered into, whereas the purpose of the midwife–woman relationship is to give and receive good midwifery care (Pairman 2000). On the other hand, the term 'partnership' may be described as 'working together towards a common aim' (Freeman *et al.* 2004, p.8). In a partnership both participants ideally have equal status, sharing power and control (Pairman 2000).

There are times when the midwife–woman partnership may be unequal. This may occur when the midwives' personal and professional project of birth and women's choices cause conflict, or when the woman makes decisions which the midwife regards as detrimental to her health, or to that of the fetus. This may challenge the balance of the midwife–woman relationship. Participants in the study suggested that the expert is able to negotiate this conflict through facilitating a trusting birth environment, valuing and supporting women's choices, and through establishing trusting relationships with women, their families and colleagues. Experts were valued for their positive characteristics, that facilitated emotional support. Supportive techniques were also suggested to facilitate the relationship. These may be physical or emotional, and include high-touch, hands-on midwifery practices or providing warmth, nurturing, gentleness, kindness, caring and positive encouragement (Kennedy 2000; Sleutel 2000; Berg & Dahlberg 2001; Lundgren & Dahlberg 2002; James *et al.* 2003).

This connection can be demonstrated physically or through the medium of 'presencing' (Kennedy 2002; Kennedy *et al.* 2004). This refers to ways of 'being there' or 'being with' another (Heidegger 1962; Nelms 1996; Benner 2001). It is a process that is characterised by sensitivity, intimacy, holism, and an adaptation to unique circumstances (Finfield-Connett 2006). It includes the capacity to guide and encourage, creating an unobtrusive environment of safety and calm (Anderson 2000). In her exploration of nursing expertise, Benner (2001) identifies presencing as an important aspect of the helping role, and therefore an important aspect of nursing expertise. Kennedy used the term 'engaged presence' to describe the essence of the relationship or the 'connection' the expert midwife has with the woman. The following quote from the study captures the essence of 'engaged presence' or 'connected presence'.

> *I sat back and watched her do what her body told her to do, and she got into whatever position she felt like and laboured very normally, very quickly, very nicely, very normal delivery and I did nothing only occasional listening to the fetal heart, that was all I did and it was, it was nice that it went well. It was quite an eye opener for me, to do nothing ... but encourage and support.*
> (Group interview, consultant unit B)

However, in order to be connected, 'the midwife must first know and understand the woman, and work with her as partner in the birth process' (Downe *et al.* 2007, p.136). As previously suggested, this

connection is facilitated through continuity of care, through giving true and honest information, supporting women's choices, and facilitating a calm and trusting birth environment.

Midwife–colleague relationship

The relationships that expert midwives form with colleagues is an area that has not been widely explored in the research literature. Hunter (2005) offers one of the few analyses of this topic. She has argued that relationships with midwifery colleagues are of key importance to hospital midwives, providing the main source of feedback on individual practice. Her research has demonstrated that both verbal and non-verbal communication are important aspects of the midwife–colleague relationship.

Participants noted that, in order to facilitate positive working relationships, the expert midwife would strive to create an environment of trust. This was facilitated through teamwork, collaborative relationships, a relaxed atmosphere and approach, and advocacy and support. Teamwork was seen to be a significant element of the care environment. It included interaction between midwives, doctors, managers and the women themselves. Effective teamwork depended on a relationship built on mutual respect and trust, and it was reported to be an essential element in a supportive birth environment.

Participants reported that experts 'nurture newly qualified staff', providing encouragement and support. They created a supported environment conducive to learning, where colleagues felt comfortable to ask questions. Experts were willing to share their knowledge, experiences and expertise, and valued the experiences, knowledge and skills of others. They were willing to learn, and identified limitations in their own practice. For this reason, their expertise did not always have to be 'on show'. They were confident in their own ability to stand back and let others take the lead.

Creating an environment of trust

> *A skilled and sensitive midwife can create an unobtrusive atmosphere of safety and calm, which allows women to feel secure enough to just disconnect mind from body . . . An intrusive midwife can just as easily block a woman's being able to do this, undermine her confidence in her own body and turn her experience of giving birth into a nightmare.*
>
> (Anderson 2000, p.117)

Participants suggested that a supportive environment is built on a foundation of mutual trust between health professionals themselves, and between midwives and labouring women. As noted above, experts demonstrated the ability to facilitate a relaxed atmosphere, and thus create an environment of co-operation and trust where colleagues were able to ask questions and learn from each other. This environment was seen to be of benefit to both women and midwives, in that it allowed expertise to develop, and it facilitated a cycle of empowerment.

However, participants acknowledged that time constraints and other environmental factors, such as poor staffing, can have a negative effect on these relationships, and thus on the birth environment. The unique philosophies, characteristics, skills and attitudes of the midwife may also play a significant role in shaping the birth environment. Participants suggested that differing philosophies caused disharmony in the working environment, and may influence birth outcomes. Those who have a fundamental distrust of birth can transfer this distrust to colleagues and to women themselves. In contrast, those midwives who fundamentally trust the normalcy of birth, and trust women's ability to give birth, strive to provide a specific kind of space in which women can birth their babies.

Similar findings were found in a study conducted by Kennedy and colleagues (2004), where the expert was suggested to 'orchestrate labour', thus creating a safe space for the woman to give birth. This safe environment appears to be underpinned by the expert's fundamental trust in birth, trust in the woman's ability to give birth, and support of women's choices. Participants in this study identified that one characteristic of expert practice was the ability to negotiate these challenges to facilitate a positive birth environment.

Summary of findings relating to connected companionship

This section has explored aspects of the connected relationship that expert midwives establish with women and their colleagues, and the techniques they use to facilitate the right environment in which these relationships can flourish. Participants noted that experts create an environment of trust through collaborative relationships with colleagues, and with childbearing women. This contributed to an environment characterised by a virtuous cycle of positive well-being and innovation for the team, and for the women using the service.

Synthesis of the findings

The four themes identified (wisdom, skilled practice, enacted vocation and connected companionship) can be synthesised into three domains of expert midwifery practice: physiological expertise, technical expertise and integrated expertise.

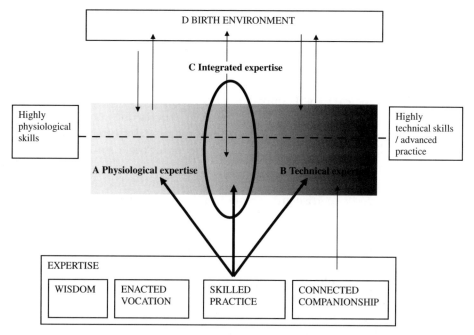

Figure 6.1 Domains of midwifery expertise. (A) Expert who demonstrates expertise in normal childbirth only. (B) Expert who demonstrates technical brilliance and is highly skilled in using equipment and birth technology. (C) Integrated expert. Strives to promote normal birth but is competent in using birth technology. Able to demonstrate expertise in high-risk and low-risk settings, and practises the same regardless of clinical environment. (D) Birth environment. Influenced by all three domains of expertise. In turn, the environment affects the capacity of midwives with technical and physiological expertise, but not integrated expertise.

As represented by Figure 6.1, the four key themes of 'wisdom', 'skilled practice', 'enacted vocation' and 'connected companionship' are fundamental to expertise. It appears to be the level of skilled practice that determines the specific domain of expertise. At one end of the spectrum, there appear to be 'experts in high-risk childbirth'. These experts have been defined as 'technical experts', characterised by their ability to display technical brilliance, being highly skilled in using equipment and birth technology. The extreme pole of technical expertise has been defined as 'advanced practice or highly technical'. These skills include more specialised practice such as performing ventouse deliveries. At the other end of the spectrum, there appear to be 'experts in normal childbirth'. These experts have been defined as 'physiological experts', mainly working at home or in birth centres. In this study, 'integrated experts' were most commonly described by participants as being characterised by the ability to demonstrate expertise in high-risk and low-risk settings, transcending their expert skills through boundaries of normality and pathology.

Separate from but also alongside the domains of expertise is the clinical environment. Both the 'technical expert' and 'physiological expert' appear to influence and be influenced by the birth environment. In other words, those who are regarded as technical experts only demonstrate specific areas of expertise evident in a technical setting. Physiological experts only demonstrate expertise in a low-risk setting. In contrast, the practice of 'integrated' experts does not appear to be influenced or affected by the birth environment. Indeed, they may act as catalysts in transforming the environment for other staff and for child-bearing women.

These three topics of technical expertise, physiological expertise and integrated expertise are explored in the next section.

Technical experts

Participants alluded to a type of expertise which was specific to high-risk childbirth. Technical experts demonstrated technical brilliance and were skilled in using equipment and birth technology. Their skills are honed and developed over time and with practice, particularly in relation to technology and equipment. It is evident in practice and in the literature that the role, skills and boundaries of midwifery practice have become expanded, extended and developed (Daly & Carnwell 2003). Midwives are now adopting roles such as ventouse practitioners and midwife ultrasonographers, and undertaking extended skills such as intravenous cannulation, which were previously conducted by medical practitioners (Lavender 2007). Terms such as advanced practice, higher-level practice or specialist practice have been used to describe the expansion of the midwife's role. Advanced midwifery practice may be defined as adjusting the boundaries for the development of future practice. Specialist practice appears to be more specific, demonstrating higher levels of knowledge and judgement in a specific area of practice (Durgahee 2003). The term 'specialist' may be defined as 'someone who has a lot of experience, knowledge or skill in a particular subject' and a technologist as 'someone who works with a particular technology' (Cambridge Online Dictionary[4]). Thus, experts in high-risk care are specialist in their knowledge and skill attributed to high-risk intrapartum care, and in using birth technology.

Technical experts were suggested to influence the birth environment, and be influenced by the birth environment. It may be argued that technical experts would not demonstrate expertise if they were taken out of the high-risk setting. This would equate to the theories of Ericsson and others working in the cognitive school of expertise (Chase &

[4] Available at: http://dictionary.cambridge.org/.

Simon 1973; Ericsson 1996; Ericsson & Smith 1991). This hypothesis requires further exploration in future studies.

Physiological experts

Experts in low-risk or normal childbirth appear to be characterised by their ability to promote normal childbirth practices in specific low-risk settings, such as at home or in birthing centres. Although experts in low-risk childbirth were seen to be competent in using equipment and following protocols within a hospital setting, they demonstrated expertise predominantly in a low-risk setting, such as the community, or birth centres.

The integration from community to hospital ways of working often requires practitioners to be able to navigate different philosophies and practices of care. Such a move has been cited by authors as a source of emotional stress for midwives (McFarlane & Downe 1999; Shallow 2001; Hunter 2004, 2005, 2006). Although not spontaneously suggested by participants, it is possible that the practice, confidence and competence of physiological experts are influenced by the birth environment, which essentially differentiates them from the 'integrated' expert. This fits with the perspective of Benner and Tanner (1987) who argue that experts can only function as experts in their own specialist areas. However, again, this hypothesis requires further testing in future studies. Practitioners in this field again demonstrate virtuoso characteristics, but in this case they seem to be allied with a strong vocational attachment to the promotion of physiological labour and birth.

Integrated experts

Benner and Tanner (1987) suggest that experts can only function as experts in their own specialist areas. While this seemed to be the case for those with technological and physiological expertise, participants in the study were more likely to describe experts who had the capacity to move fluidly between a range of environments. They could also work effectively with women with straightforward pregnancies and births, and those who had complex problems. This domain is termed 'integrated expertise'. We reached the following synthesis, based on the findings from both the meta-synthesis and the data collection with midwives:

The integrated expert possesses the essential personal characteristics, and demonstrates the necessary skill and ability to promote normal childbirth, to recognise deviations from the norm and to use technological interventions appropriately in order to facilitate optimal birth outcomes for childbearing women, and to fulfil the emotional, physical and spiritual needs of the woman and her family in any setting. Integrated experts respond dynamically to a range of settings, positively influencing the setting and those working within it.

The characteristics of integrated experts are strongly aligned with those of the adaptive expert discussed in Chapter 5 (Hatano & Inagaki 1986). There are also affective elements in the mix, suggesting that affect theory (Tomkins 1991) might be a useful underpinning for this kind of expertise. Affect theory proposes that emotions are hardwired to biological reactions. This would suggest that so-called 'illness scripts' (Schmidt & Rikers 2007) or possibly, in the case of physiological labour and birth, 'wellness scripts', that arise from incidents that evoke strong emotional reactions are particularly likely to be coded into the memory in chunks. It may be that adaptive (integrated) experts are exhibiting high levels of emotional intelligence, and are particularly adept at linking the biological impact of particular emotions to these memory chunks (Chase & Simon 1973), making them easier to access and use in similar situations.

Conclusion

Data from the studies described in this chapter identified three domains of expert midwifery practice: physiological expertise, technological expertise and integrated expertise. In the interviews, characteristics of integrated expertise were reported more often than those of either technical or physiological expertise. Integrated experts appear to transcend the boundaries of normality and pathology, negotiating the pull between the active management and expectant management of labour, and successfully navigating the dichotomy between the medical and holistic models of care. They exhibited characteristics that were strongly aligned with the theories of adaptive expertise (Hatano & Inagaki 1986), and of affect (Tomkins 1991).

Physiological expertise and technical expertise appear to be two distinct paradigms at opposite ends of a continuum, each with a distinct repertoire (Schön 1983). At each end, experts demonstrate particular skills in either low- or high-risk care, with the practitioners' ability to demonstrate this expertise being influenced by the clinical environment in which they work. This appears to be an important characteristic that differentiates them from integrated experts.

Four main themes (wisdom, skilled practice, enacted vocation and connected companionship) were identified as fundamental components of intrapartum maternity care expertise. The hypothesis generated by the data suggests that all expert intrapartum maternity care practitioners will demonstrate particular aspects of these components. The findings also suggest that the expert intrapartum practitioners encountered by the midwife participants were courageous, demonstrated leadership qualities, and were successful in their ability to motivate, encourage and inspire others. Using experts as role models may be an effective way of improving practice, challenging cultural norms, and promoting evidence-based care. Future research in this area might usefully address theories of expertise from both cognitive psychology and from phenomenology, to develop approaches to recognising and encouraging the development of integrated, adaptive expertise in maternity care.

References

Alexander J (1993) Degrees in midwifery: aspirations and reality. *Journal of Advanced Nursing* 18:339–42.

Allen D (2004) Ethnomethodological insights into insider–outsider relationships in nursing ethnographies of health care settings. *Nursing Inquiry* 11(1): 14–24.

Anderson T (2000) Feeling safe enough to let go: the relationship between a woman and her midwife during the second stage of labour. In Kirkham M (ed) *The Midwife–Mother Relationship*. Basingstoke, Macmillan, 92–118.

Ang B (2002) The quest for nursing excellence. *Singapore Medical Journal* 43(10): 493.

Annendale EC (1998) How midwives accomplish natural birth: managing risk and balancing expectations. *Social Problems* 35(2): 95–110.

Ardelt M (2004) Wisdom as expert knowledge system: a critical review of a contemporary operationalization of an ancient concept. *Human Development* 47:257–85.

Barwise C (1998) Episiotomy and decision making. *British Journal of Midwifery* 6 (12): 787–90.

Baylor A (1997) A three-component conception of intuition: immediacy, sensing relationships, and reason. *New Ideas in Psychology* 15(2): 185–94.

Benner P (2001) *From Novice to Expert. Excellence and Power in Clinical Nursing Practice*. Commemorative edition. New Jersey, Prentice-Hall.

Benner P, Tanner C (1987) Clinical judgment: how expert nurses use intuition. *American Journal of Nursing* 87:23–31.

Berg M, Dahlberg K (2001) Swedish midwives' care of women who are at high obstetric risk, or who have obstetric complications. *Midwifery* 17:59–66.

Calvert S (2002) Being with women. The midwife–woman relationship. In Mander R, Fleming V (eds) *Failure to Progress. The Contraction of the Midwifery Profession*. London, Routledge.

Chase WG, Simon HA (1973) The mind's eye in chess. In Chase WG (ed) *Visual Information Processing*. New York, Academic Press, 215–81.

Cioffi J, Markham R (1997) Clinical decision making by midwives: managing case complexities. *Journal of Advanced Nursing* 25:265–72.

Clancy T (2003) Courage and today's nurse leader. *Nursing Administration* 27(2): 128–32.

Coster S, Redfern S, Wilson–Barnett SJ, Evans A, Peccei R, Guest D (2006) Impact of the role of nurse, midwife and health visitor consultant. *Journal of Advanced Nursing* 55(3): 352–63.

Daly W, Carnwell R (2003) Nursing roles and levels of practice: a framework for differentiating between elementary, specialist and advancing nursing practice. *Journal of Clinical Nursing* 12:158–67.

Davis-Floyd R (1996) Intuition as authoritative knowledge in midwifery and homebirth. *Medical Anthropology Quarterly* 10(2): 237–69.

Downe S, Simpson L, Trafford K (2007) Expert intrapartum care: a meta-synthesis. *Journal of Advanced Nursing* 57(2): 127–40.

Dreyfus HL, Dreyfus SE (1986) *Mind Over Machine. The Power of Human Intuition and Expertise in the Era of the Computer*. Oxford, Blackwell.

Dreyfus SE (2004) The five stage model of adult skill acquisition. *Bulletin of Science, Technology and Society*. http://bst.sagepub.com/cgi/content/abstract/24/3/177 (accessed June, 2010).

Durgahee, T (2003) Higher level practice: degree or specialist practice? *Nurse Education Today* 23:191–201.

Eraut M (1994) *Developing Professional Knowledge and Competence*. London, Falmer Press.

Ericsson KA (ed) (1996) *The Road to Excellence: The Acquisition of Expert Performance in the Arts and Sciences, Sports, and Games*. Mahwah, NJ, Erlbaum.

Ericsson KA, Smith J (eds) (1991) *Toward a General Theory of Expertise: Prospects and Limits*. Cambridge, Cambridge University Press.

Finfield-Connett D (2006) Metasynthesis of presence in nursing. *Journal compilation*. Oxford, Blackwell, 708–14.

Fleming VE (1998) Women-with-midwives-with-women: a model of interdependence. *Midwifery* 14:137–43.

Fleming V, Milde J (2000) Cultural learning: midwifery in Scotland and Germany. *British Journal of Midwifery* 8(6): 368–73.

Freeman L, Timperley H, Adair V (2004) Partnership in midwifery care in New Zealand. *Midwifery* 20:2–14.

Gould D (2004) Trust me, I am a midwife. *British Journal of Midwifery* 12(1): 44.

Harbison J (2000) Clinical decision making in nursing: theoretical perspectives and their relevance to practice. *Journal of Advanced Nursing* 35(1): 126–33.

Hatano G, Inagaki K (1986) Two courses of expertise. *Child Development and Education in Japan* 262–72.

Heidegger M (1962) *Being and Time*. New York, Harper and Row.

Heischman D (2002) Moral courage. *Teaching and School Leadership* 62(1).

Henderson A (1969) Excellence in nursing. *American Journal of Nursing* 69(9): 2133.

Humphreys A, Johnson S, Richardson J, Stenhouse E, Watkin M (2007) A systematic review and meta-synthesis: evaluating the effectiveness of nurse, midwife/allied health professional consultants. *Journal of Clinical Nursing* 16:1792–808.

Hunter B (2004) Conflicting ideologies as a source of emotion work in midwifery. *Midwifery* 20:261–72.

Hunter B (2005) Emotion work and boundary maintenance in hospital-based midwifery. *Midwifery* 21:253–66.

Hunter B (2006) The importance of reciprocity in relationships between community based midwives' and mothers. *Midwifery* 22:308–22.

International Confederation of Midwives (2005) Definition of a midwife. www. internationalmidwives.org/Documentation/Coredocuments/tabid/322/ Default.aspx (accessed June, 2010).

James DC, Simpson KR, Knox GE (2003) How do expert labor nurses view their role? *Journal of Obstetric, Gynecological and Neonatal Nursing* 32(6): 814–23.

Kennedy HP (2000) A model of exemplary midwifery practice: results of a Delphi study. *Journal of Midwifery and Women's Health* 45(1): 4–19.

Kennedy HP (2002) The midwife as an 'instrument' of care. *American Journal of Public Health* 92(11): 1759–60.

Kennedy HP, Shannon MT, Chuahorn U, Kravetz K (2004) The landscape of caring for women: a narrative study of midwifery practice. *Journal of Midwifery and Women's Health* 49(1): 14–23.

Kennedy M (1987) Inexact sciences: professional education and the development of expertise. *Review of Research in Education* 14:133–67.

King L, Appleton J (1997) Intuition: a critical review of the research and rhetoric. *Journal of Advanced Nursing* 26:194–202.

Kirkham M (ed) (2000) *The Midwife–Woman Relationship.* Basingstoke, Macmillan.

Lauder W (1994) Beyond reflection, practice wisdom and the practical syllogism. *Nurse Education Today* 14(2): 91–8.

Lavender T (2007) New roles for midwives. *British Journal of Midwifery* 15(1): 6.

Litchfield M (1999) Practice wisdom. *Advanced Nursing Science* 22(2): 62–73.

Lundgren I, Dahlberg K (2002) Midwives' experience of the encounter with women and their pain during childbirth. *Midwifery* 18(2): 155–64.

Macleod Clark J, Maben J, Jones K (2009) Project 2000: perceptions of the philosophy and practice of nursing: shifting perceptions – a new practitioner? *Journal of Advanced Nursing* 26(1): 161–8.

Mavroidis C (2003) A partnership in courage. *Society of Thoracic Surgeons* 75:1366–471.

McFarlane S, Downe S (1999) An interpretation of midwives' views about the nature of midwifery. *Practising Midwife* 2(11): 23–6.

Nelms T (1996) Living a caring presence in nursing: a Heideggerian hermeneutical analysis. *Journal of Advanced Nursing* 24:368–74.

Newble D (1992) Assessing clinical competence at the undergraduate level. *Medical Education* 26(6): 503–11.

Pairman S (2000) Women-centred midwifery: partnerships or professional friendship? In Kirkham M (ed) *The Midwife–Woman Relationship.* Basingstoke, Macmillan, 207–25.

Rew L (1990) Intuition in critical care nursing practice. *Dimensions of Critical Care Nursing* 9(1): 30–7.

Salvage J (2004) The call to nurture. *Nursing Standard* 19(10): 16–17.

Schmidt HG, Rikers RM (2007) How expertise develops in medicine: knowledge encapsulation and illness script formation. *Medical Education* 41(12): 1133–9.

Schön D (1983) *The Reflective Practitioner. How Professionals Think in Action.* London, Temple Smith.

Shallow H (2001) Competence and confidence: working in a climate of fear. *British Journal of Midwifery* 9(4): 237–44.

Shapiro MM (1998) A career ladder based on Benner's model: an analysis of expected outcomes. *Journal of Nursing Administration* 28(3): 13–19.

Sleutel M (2000) Intrapartum nursing care: a case study of supportive interventions and ethical conflicts. *Birth* 27(1): 38–45.

Thorstensen K (2000) Trusting women, essential to midwifery. *Journal of Midwifery and Women's Health* 45(5): 405–7.

Tomkins S (1991) *Affect Imagery Consciousness: Anger and Fear,* vol 3. New York, Springer.

Tritten J (1992) Giving voice to wisdom (editorial). *Midwifery Today* 23:1.

Truman P (2002) Use your intuition. *Nursing Standard* 16(34): 23.

Walsh D (1999) An ethnographic study of women's experience of partnership caseload midwifery practice: the professional as a friend. *Midwifery* 15(3): 165–76.

White K (2002) Nursing as vocation. *Nursing Ethics* 9(3): 279–90.

Woodward V (1997) Professional caring: a contradiction in terms? *Journal of Advanced Nursing* 26:999–1004.

Worth-Butler M, Murphy R, Fraser D (1995) The need to define competence in midwifery. *British Journal of Midwifery* 3(15): 259–62.

Wright S (2004) Say goodbye. *Nursing Standard* 18(34): 22–3.

Young CE (1987) Intuition and nursing processes. *Holistic Nursing Practice* 1(3): 52–62.

Chapter 7
Enhancing Expertise and Skills Through Education

Denis Walsh

Introduction

One of the striking differences between midwifery and obstetric journals is their approach to the care of childbearing women. The journals of midwifery are replete with what might be called broadly psychosocial approaches examining attitudes, emotions and interpersonal relationships while the latter focus on the clinical aspects of care such as pathologies, screening, diagnostics and treatment. Underpinning both approaches are the more elusive ideas of expertise, competence and skills. After all, no woman would want to be looked after by a robotic carer who could diagnose and treat problems but could not communicate, nor by a compassionate carer without knowledge and assessment capabilities. The effective professional is someone who can marry both knowledge and caring behaviours.

Over the past 10 years I have been running workshops around evidence for normal birth. My preoccupation at the start was to address the knowledge deficit that I thought was afflicting midwifery practice. Over the last 2 years, I have added a skills workshop in normal birth to address the need for effective application of knowledge. This workshop engages much more with attitudes and philosophies of care.

During the evolution of these sessions, I have come to realise that expertise incorporates a range of factors. In this chapter I will discuss the development of my own understanding of expertise against the backdrop of the educational events I have been running for midwives all over the UK, and in parts of Europe, Australia and New Zealand.

Essential Midwifery Practice: Leadership, Expertise and Collaborative Working, first edition. Edited by Soo Downe, Sheena Byrom and Louise Simpson
Published 2011 by Blackwell Publishing Ltd.
© 2011 Blackwell Publishing Ltd.

The context for normal birth workshops

My midwifery training took place within a largely biomedical paradigm. In my early years of practice, I had a growing unease about how childbirth was conducted in large maternity hospitals. In the late 1990s, I was working as a research and development midwife in a large consultant unit. I was becoming increasingly aware that significant amounts of evidence in support of normal labour and birth were not recognised or implemented. I began to compile evidence in these areas. This process eventually morphed into ten sessions of teaching, covering most areas of labour and birth practice. Broadly, the sessions covered the topics of birth environment; first-stage labour progress, spontaneous rupture of membranes and feeding in labour; posture and positions; fetal heart monitoring; progress in labour; pain relief in labour; care of the perineum; the third stage of labour; and changing practice. The sessions comprised summary presentations of evidence in each of these areas, followed by group work.

After advertising the evidence course, I had a steady stream of bookings across the UK to run it. This turned into around 20 courses a year over the next 8 years. I always did evaluations, and these were generally very positive. Very rarely, I received emails some weeks later from midwives who had attended the course, speaking of how they had rediscovered their enthusiasm for their work. However, I was increasingly uneasy that simply imparting knowledge to midwives was not necessarily changing practice.

Attitudes and beliefs

During the period of 2002 to 2005, I completed a PhD on the birth centre model and, in the course of reading and writing for this, I became aware of how attitudes and beliefs shape practice. Studying a small free-standing birth centre also reminded me how much the context of care also influenced practice. In 2004, a midwife colleague told me a striking story, about another midwife she had worked with some years earlier. She was a community midwife who enjoyed attending home births. On one occasion, a baby was born unexpectedly unresponsive. It was transferred to the nearest neonatal unit and subsequently developed cerebral palsy. The midwife was devastated, taking some time off for stress before returning to community practice. My colleague went on to say that she met a pregnant woman at the school gates some time later who told her of a curious conversation she had had with her community midwife about home birth. At the booking interview, she asked the midwife about her attitude to home birth as she had been considering it with this baby. The midwife replied: `I am not for it, and I am not against it´. The woman concluded that she was against and never broached the subject again. My colleague asked the woman the name of the midwife. It was the midwife who had experienced the unresponsive baby. Later, my colleague discovered that this midwife had not attended a home birth since that experience. This is a sad tale of how birth experiences can profoundly affect subsequent practice.

I took the opportunity to examine my own attitudes towards birth when I came across an exercise suggested by Mavis Kirkham called personal construct laddering (Kirkham 1995). This asks you to brainstorm thoughts and ideas that come to you when presented with a phrase like: *What I believe about labour and birth is …* Through this exercise I became aware of just how seminal the attendance of my own children's birth had been, and how they shaped my subsequent practice. Our second daughter was a water birth and a wonderful experience. I have been a big fan of water birth ever since. One useful trigger to help midwives reflect on attitudes and beliefs is to ask them to recall special births that they attended as a midwife that stay in the memory. The one that came to my mind was attending a water birth at home of a 39-year-old woman with a history of ME. I recall it in some detail below to demonstrate the powerful effect it had on me.

I did all Sally's antenatal care at her home and observed over the course of the pregnancy a remission in her symptoms of ME. She was genuinely excited about the baby and birth and went into labour on a bright sunny morning in July. After a reasonably quick first stage and a tiring 2-hour second stage, she gave birth to a robust baby girl in the pool. It was a magical moment. The conservatory doors to the garden were open, the sun was streaming through and we could hear children playing in the adjacent neighbour's garden during the labour. She did not lack energy during the labour, she pushed with great gusto, and her and partner were ecstatic at the birth. She was a confident, instinctive mother. I remember driving home after the birth, feeling proud and elated that I had facilitated a birth that I am sure would have been interventionist in a maternity hospital. In the late 1990s, an elderly primigravida with a history of a chronic, debilitating condition would not have been seen as a good candidate for a home birth.

For me, it was the realisation of an ideal regarding what being a midwife was all about: personalised, supportive, empathic care for a woman according to her needs and her choices. I had not witnessed a medical event, but one of nature's marvels – human childbirth in the perfect setting. She had done it, and I was the privileged bystander. To this day, I understand her experience as a healing one. The tentative, introspective woman she was at the beginning of pregnancy grew into a strong, confident mother. She had gone on a transformatory journey and it was beautiful to witness. After such an experience, it is no surprise that I have been a strong believer in home birth ever since.

Birth environment

In the main, UK midwives work within large hospital settings. There is evidence that they struggle to reconcile their beliefs about birth when working within this setting. Blaaka and Eri (2008) capture this tension in their insightful phenomenological account of seven midwives' descriptions of skilled midwifery in a Norwegian high-technology labour ward. They conclude that midwives are doing midwifery between two belief systems and that a power struggle between these two belief systems is played out in the birth room. Their reflection is reminiscent of Machin and Scamell's (1997) paper which captured this tension in the phrase the `irresistible nature of the biomedical metaphor´ where women who were orientated to and desiring of a normal birth when pregnant went on to embrace technology and intervention when confronted with the labour experience on a highly technological labour ward.

Exposure to a radical alternative can be the catalyst for attitudinal change. When I first observed care in a birth centre, I was confronted with a completely different approach to time in labour. Midwives had time to simply be with women and there was no pressure to process them through an assembly-line birthing model (Walsh 2006). These ideas of altered temporality around birth are explored in depth in Brown and Chandra's (2009) thought-provoking paper `Slow midwifery´, highlighting midwifery presence as a key mediator of therapeutic benefit. Midwifery presence is an important theme in literature around expertise in midwifery. Pembroke and Pembroke (2008) summarise the literature, stating that presence is to do with the quality of the relationship between midwife and woman, with altruism and self-giving and with building trust and confidence. Byrom and Downe (2008) suggest that emotional intelligence is a hallmark of expertise, grounding it in relationships.

All these authors highlight the conditions where midwifery therapeutic presence will be expressed and developed. Non-medical birth settings provide such a context. The birth environment can be a powerful catalyst for changing attitudes.

Enhancing skills for normal labour and birth

As already mentioned, I began to question whether simply sharing knowledge about the considerable evidence in support of normal birth was enough to change practice. There were a few missing links between knowledge and its implementation via skills and attitudes. For these reasons I decided to develop a course that examined attitudes and skills in promoting normality. In addition, I built into the course an exercise that required participants to plan and implement a practice change, based on the course materials and the learning they had acquired.

Making a personal birth philosophy explicit can be assisted by exposure to literature on models of care. Much has been written about the contrasting midwifery/social and biomedical models of care (Davis-Floyd 1992; Wagner 1994) and, at their best, these texts highlight important differences of emphasis between these approaches. However, some of the literature in this area can imply, or even state, that individuals can be neatly allocated to medical or midwifery ways of practising. This increasingly predictable dichotomy is becoming hackneyed and `tired´. Fresh language is needed to move the debate on. The Midwives Association of North America (MANA) provides an alternative with its philosophy of care, reported on by Davis-Floyd and Davis (1997). Box 7.1 sets out the key principles of childbirth for members of MANA. When I present this list as a slide at the beginning of the skills course, I have noted first a curiosity and then, in some midwives, a dawning of awareness – like a light being switched on that brings clarity and purpose. This is often reflected in comments on the evaluation forms. Here is the sample from the last 2 years.

Box 7.1 Midwives' creed (from the Midwives' Association of North America)

Childbirth is about:

- women as creators
- oneness between mother and baby
- power, beauty, strength of woman's body in birth
- mother's intuitive knowledge of herself and her baby
- a sense of mystery around birth
- a rites of passage experience
- transformation and opportunity for personal growth
- being symbolised by love, not fear

I came here today on the brink of giving up midwifery, but then remembered what I love about my profession and why I was drawn to it all those years ago – it was the MANA's midwives' creed . . .

For the last 5 years I have been coasting in the system, not really enjoying it but not yet burnt out. The philosophy exercise helped me to realise that I have been working with a `glass half empty´ attitude and to think how enthusiastic I was when I first qualified . . .

> I have never really recovered from a terrible experience a couple of years ago when I delivered a fresh stillbirth. Working outside a high tech labour ward has scared me ever since. However, I now feel ready to face that again, after all it was why I came into midwifery. That birth philosophy is still down deep inside me. I realised that today.

Articulating a philosophy of birth is personal and even private. I observe some midwives writing on to a second page. Some appear to write very little. I don't ask them to share their thoughts because I judge that it might prevent them from being honest and open. At the end of 2 days, it is clear that the course itself has an unambiguous underlying set of beliefs. Comments on how individuals have been affected are more numerous after 2 days than just 1 day. One of the pioneers of birth workshops, Andrea Robertson (1997), made this observation early on in her career and began to run 2-day events to maximise their effects. She also told me how to spot when course materials have `got under someone's skin´. If, in the midst of excellent evaluations, there is a rogue one, then this can indicate that the person had been challenged. Over the years, I have noticed that particular comments may point to this. For example: `disappointed, learn nothing I have not heard before´, `these approaches don't work with women who attend our hospital´. Commonly, the comment `thought-provoking´ is recorded which indicates a willingness to examine alternative approaches and indicates that midwives are considering changes.

Expertise and group work

If the philosophy exercise prompts an individual midwife to examine beliefs, then group work facilitates what that might mean for actual practice. After each presentation that summarises up-to-date evidence, midwives gather in groups to share experiences and ideas around the topic area. This is where stories are swapped and practices discussed. Michael Polanyi (1969) provides an illuminating insight into how people accrue knowledge and skills. Polanyi, a Swiss chemist, wrote of people learning through observing connoisseurs and experts and then copying what they have seen. This is the master/apprentice model. He called this learning `personal knowledge´ and it applies well to midwifery. Personal learning is the learning of student midwives observing and mimicking their midwifery mentors. It is the learning of newly qualified midwives being preceptored in their early years. It is also the knowledge accrued through reflecting on practice with another colleague.

Feedback on the group work often highlights that midwives had no idea there was such variation in practice between hospitals. It opens their eyes to alternatives, especially if they work within an institutional setting. Issues like flexibility with access to water birth, the commonness of physiological third stage and home assessment in early labour are just a few examples. The following comments capture some of this.

> I was amazed to hear that their anaesthetists are recommending water birth prior to considering an epidural.

> I have not seen a physiological third stage in 8 years of full-time practice and they are having them every day.

> This newly qualified midwife said she had rarely seen a `hands on´ birth but I have rarely seen a `hands off´ one.

> I can't imaging how they (*other staff*) would respond if we took the bed out of the room but they don't even have a bed in their birth centre to start with . . .

Systematic reviews of strategies that have successfully influenced changes in practice indicate that interactive group discussions can be effective (O'Brien *et al*. 2008). The groups have to be small, no more than six or seven. They work better when participants have varied experiences, and when they have focused questions to consider. As the focus of the course is skills for normal labour and birth, higher level skills are exercised in *keeping birth normal* (my emphasis) when labour moves into the grey area between normality and abnormality. For this reason, a number of real case scenarios are presented to the groups that challenge them to consider what they would do if faced with them. Scenarios are minimalist to prompt creative thinking. After discussion within the group, they feedback to the larger group and then the real outcome is revealed. Further discussion ensues.

This approach is premised on problem-based learning (Wood 2003), now widely used in training for the health professions, including midwifery. It enables practitioners to apply decision making within the complexities of practice and to think through the application of knowledge to a unique individual. This is the artistry of practice, an elusive concept that some believe is being lost with the advent of evidential guidelines and algorithms (Greatbatch *et al*. 2005; Hunter & Segrott 2008).

Audit project

The final session on the 2-day skills course requires the midwives to work with their fellow midwives from the same maternity unit, with the aim of deciding on a mini-project that they will take back to practice. This approach is based on change management research, which found that local consensus processes of getting representatives of various groups to sign up to a project can be effective in bringing about results (O'Brien *et al.* 2008). It harnesses the power of `bottom-up´ initiatives. The structure the groups follow is:

- identify and agree on an issue from practice
- identify barriers to change
- decide on strategies to address the barriers
- define a time frame for bringing about change
- identify how to measure the change.

These steps roughly follow Kulier *et al.*'s (2008) recommendations of moving from evidence to effect.

- Knowledge and awareness
- Acceptance and persuasion (addressing barriers)
- Decision making (strategies)
- Implementation (time frame)
- Continuation (measuring outcomes)

Over the years, a whole variety of projects have been suggested from this exercise, including removing beds from birth rooms, implementing a triage facility for labour admissions, addressing skills for physiological third stage, adapting the partogram to make it more flexible, restructuring antenatal education to make it more effective, and increasing the uptake of water birth.

Arguably, the most crucial stage in this cycle is the last one. I always request midwives to email me at a later date with outcomes from these plans. My expectations are not high for a widespread response to this request, but many of those I do receive indicate that attendance can influence practice change, as is evident in the examples below.

> Over the last 3 months our water birth rate has steadily increased and at least now a few of us are committed to moving that on.

> We had our first case last week of a primip going into water for slow labour and guess what – she had a water birth!!! Even the obstetricians were talking about it.

> We have increased our physiological third stage rate but now at the monthly review, people are saying we must be coercing women into it because the unit policy is not to recommend it. Any advice . . .

The key to embedding new practices is in the ongoing commitment of those present and, from that perspective, the impact of a one-off 2-day training event is limited. However, the adjustment made over the years to the original evidence course has resulted in more anecdotal feedback that its impact lasts beyond the actual time of attendance.

Conclusion

Addressing the area of midwifery expertise by focusing on training, courses and workshops is one strategy and should not be seen in isolation from other initiatives. Byrom and Downe (2008) highlight the importance of transformational leadership in affecting change. Downe *et al.* (2007) concluded that wisdom, skilled practice and enacted vocation contribute to our understanding of midwifery expertise, El-Nemer *et al.* (2006) talk about `skilled help from the heart´, Berg (2005) writes of `genuine caring in caring for the genuine´ and Price and Johnson (2006) prefer artistry to expertise, noting its tacit nature and its emotional content. All these authors write about expertise, and hint at what can facilitate and nurture its expression, without really fleshing out the definitive steps to guarantee its acquisition. No doubt that is because it is multidimensional and complex, as illustrated in the previous chapters in this section. More research is needed in this area, and into strategies that maximise the development of effective midwifery expertise. Specifically, the experiences described in this chapter indicate that a course of targeted training and education that is based on theories of transformation and change can address key aspects that are known to make a difference, even over the short period of 2 days. These include practitioners' beliefs, the context of practice, and the power of small groups to both creatively solve problems in particular clinical scenarios and plan a `do-able´ project for long-term practice change.

References

Berg M (2005) A midwifery model of care for childbearing women at high risk: genuine caring in caring for the genuine. *Journal of Perinatal Education* 14: 9–2.

Blaaka G, Eri T (2008) Doing midwifery between different belief systems. *Midwifery* 24: 344–52.

Brown J, Chandra A (2009) Slow midwifery. *Women and Birth* 22: 29–33.

Byrom S, Downe S (2008) `She sort of shines´: midwives' accounts of `good´ midwifery and `good´ leadership. *Midwifery* 26(1): 126–37.

Davis-Floyd R (1992) *Birth as an American Rite of Passage*. London, University of California Press.

Davis-Floyd R, Davis E (1997) Intuition as authoritative knowledge in midwifery and homebirth. In Davis-Floyd R, Sargent C (eds) *Childbirth and Authoritative Knowledge*. London, University of California Press, 315–49.

Downe S, Simpson L, Trafford K (2007) Expert intrapartum maternity care: a meta-synthesis. *Journal of Advanced Nursing* 57(2): 127–40.

El-Nemer A, Downe S, Small N (2006) `She would help me from the heart´: an ethnography of Egyptian women in labour. *Social Science and Medicine* 62: 81–92.

Greatbatch D, Hanlon G, Goode J, O'Caithain A, Strangleman T, Luff D (2005) Telephone triage, expert systems and clinical expertise. *Sociology of Health and Illness* 27(6): 802–30.

Hunter B, Segrott J (2008) Re-mapping client journeys and professional identities: a review of the literature on clinical pathways. *International Journal of Nursing Studies* 45: 608–25.

Kirkham M (1995) *Using Personal Planning to Meet the Challenge of Changing Childbirth*. ENB Resource Pack 1,3. London, ENB.

Kulier R, Gee H, Khan K (2008) Five steps from evidence to effect: exercising clinical freedom to implement research findings. *British Journal of Obstetrics and Gynaecology* 115: 1197–202.

Machin D, Scamell M (1997) The experience of labour: using ethnography to explore the irresistible nature of the bio-medical metaphor during labour. *Midwifery* 13: 78–84.

O'Brien MA, Freemantle N, Oxman AD, Wolf F, Davis DA, Herrin J (2008) Continuing education meetings and workshops: effects on professional practice and health care outcomes (Cochrane Review). The Cochrane Library, Issue 1, 2008. Chichester, John Wiley.

Pembroke M, Pembroke J (2008) The spirituality of presence in midwifery care. *Midwifery* 24: 321–7.

Polanyi M (1969) *Knowing and Being*. Chicago, IL, University of Chicago.

Price M, Johnson M (2006) An ethnography of experienced midwives caring for women in labour. *Evidence Based Midwifery* 4(3): 101–6.

Robertson A (1997) *The Midwife Companion*. Sydney, Ace Graphics.

Wagner M (1994) *Pursuing the Birth Machine: the search for appropriate birth technology*. Camperdown, Australia, Ace Graphics.

Walsh D (2006) Subverting assembly-line birth: childbirth in a free-standing birth centre. *Social Science and Medicine* 62: 1330–40.

Wood D (2003) Problem based learning. *British Medical Journal* 326: 328–30.

Chapter 8
What is a Skilled Birth Attendant? Insights from South America

Ann Davenport

Introduction

I remember the first time I did a vaginal examination on a woman in labour during a 'house call' in the mountains of western Bolivia. When I turned my back to wash my hands, she ran out the door, waddled up the hill and birthed her baby in a dense cornfield. As a midwife, I had been trained to investigate, to prepare and to bring my expertise to bear on the childbearing act. How many centimetres dilated? Is it time to 'deliver' the baby? Hot water and warm towels in the room? This was her seventh baby, a baby that would be born at home, without help, and drop onto the waiting sheepskin floor cover just like the first six before him. She didn't need me telling her when it was time to give birth. Her body knew. I was the one who didn't know anything. This rural woman was shamed by me, made nervous by me, and risked her life and her baby's life by running away from me. Some midwife. Some 'expert on childbirth'.

This chapter provides a reflection on the nature of 'expertise', in the context of the issues arising from this experience.

The context of expertise

Those of us who have a university education think we know what's best for those who don't. Thanks to well-meaning people from well-developed rich countries, healthcare reform is on the agenda

Essential Midwifery Practice: Leadership, Expertise and Collaborative Working, first edition. Edited by Soo Downe, Sheena Byrom and Louise Simpson
Published 2011 by Blackwell Publishing Ltd.
© 2011 Blackwell Publishing Ltd.

everywhere, and it should be. But who is writing that agenda? Most likely, those same people who were taught inside institutions of higher learning – people who live light-years from the only mud-slick road to the health post, where the doctor is out, the pharmacy does not exist, and the next bus to a city with a hospital leaves on Wednesday.

People with university degrees in medicine, midwifery or nursing tend to see life, and especially birth, as problematic. We who have spent years surrounded by fatality, infirmity and frailty want to step in and rescue. We are *trained* to rescue. The patient (or, in most cases, the body, body part or disease) morphs into a malfunctioning machine to us, and our goal is a well-working machine. When we are sent out into the world of real women, we come armed with our good intentions, our education, our self-authority and our desire to 'make the world a better place' for these poor rural or urban or refugee women and their fly-encrusted babies. Midwives are *trained* to care.

However, in the real world with real people, in a non-medical and social/ecological model, life is a solution rather than something to be manipulated and rescued. Dr Wagner, perinatologist and public health specialist, reminds us in *Pursuing the Birth Machine* (Wagner 1994) that the most important health statistic in the world is the global mortality rate: 100%. And since we all die, the important thing is to live well. Human beings are part of a vast ecological system, one that includes both the interior and the exterior of the organism we inhabit. It includes our social status, our family and community, our support systems, our spiritual beliefs, our mental state and the physiological care we give to ourselves and each other.

Ina May Gaskin, traditional midwife, author of *Spiritual Midwifery* (Gaskin 1978) and co-founder of The Farm in Summertown, Tennessee, writes that birth is not only a biological event (anatomical, physiological and biochemical). It's also an event that transforms those who experience it and those who witness it, due to the mental and spiritual components of pregnancy and childbirth. Indispensable to this view, of course, is that birth, by nature, springs from femininity, intuition, sexuality and spirituality. All traditional midwives, and their clients, know exactly what Gaskin is talking about.

Pregnancy and childbirth say more than any other life event about the status of women in a society. Anthropologists have observed that people's belief systems underlie all fundamental practices in all cultures, particularly the rituals and taboos dealing with mating, birth and death. Modern medicine (especially obstetrics) has emerged as the new and *competing* belief system, with its own set of taboos, rituals and mysteries – belief systems that are, in a way, the hallmarks of a competing religion (Davis-Floyd 1992).

Although modern medicine has indeed saved the lives of many babies and mothers, we must remember that the most important factors for the decrease in maternal mortality and morbidity rates are not medical but social (Richmond 1990). These factors include educating girls, better nutrition, hygienic practices by doctors and contraception. Midwives know better than anyone that social factors are the connection to a healthy pregnancy and birth or a deadly one.

Health procedures and policy cannot be isolated from the larger socio-economic context in which they occur. *Poverty* – not cultural ceremony or medical ritual – contributes to poor health, and poor health contributes to poverty. Anthropologist Joan E. Paluzzi (2004) succinctly outlines in *Unhealthy Health Policy* the reasons why the World Bank's structural adjustment policies have *worsened* the quality of life among the world's poorest people. The World Bank focuses interventions and funding on single-cause/single-intervention programmes (for example, HIV prevention funding that denies sex education). The disconnection of policies and programmes from real people and real poverty has helped to increase the number of poor people suffering from interconnected health problems.

It may seem like common sense to ask a person what they want before we go about giving them what we think they need. Leave it to the anthropologists, sociologists and women birthing in cornfields to point out this obvious fact to us. Whenever we train doctors and midwives in emergency obstetric care in developing countries (sponsored by WHO and the Johns Hopkins Program for International Education in Gynaecology and Obstetrics – see their training programmes at www. jhpiego.net), the first thing the professional participants usually want to know is: when do we have the class on ultrasound or learn to manipulate the fetal monitoring machines? They are always surprised when we focus on life-saving skills using our five senses, our hands, our stethoscopes and fetoscopes, simple drugs and straightforward low-tech interventions that prevent complications and save lives. These are the types of things that most traditional midwives already know about and use. Instead of using drugs, they have an ancient and proven arsenal of medicinal plants at their disposal, along with designated body movements, ceremonial foods, and other magical gestures that their clients know and expect to receive from their midwife.

In his book about marketing social behaviour changes to influence health, Alan Andreason (1995) insists that '. . . the number one feature for influencing healthy behaviour is that consumer acceptance is the bottom line'. (Note he did not mention acceptance by the doctor, the midwife or the nurse.) Not only must social programmes be cost effective, but all strategies must begin with the client in mind. Andreason also reminds us to recognise and identify competition, and factor that into any public health policy. The most obvious competition to a normal, healthy pregnancy and birth remains cultural ritual and social values – those of the customer *and* those of the medical professionals.

As an example, the pregnant woman has the common sense and physical need to give birth in an upright position. The doctor is trained to attend a birth with the woman flat on her back, with his comfort in mind, not hers. Who wins this competition?

Integrating competition in expertise

A stark example of competition between customer acceptance and medical intervention concerns the caste system in Nepal and India. Only one caste handles blood, and that caste does not include the doctor, nurse or midwife. Health professionals may attend births (that naturally involve blood) only because they use plastic aprons, gloves and protective eye barriers to prevent the blood from touching them or vice versa. I discovered this when I spent a week in a small town in western Nepal conducting a follow-up visit for a group of midwives who had attended our training in Kathmandu earlier that month. I observed a midwife, one of our students, attending a birth with good infection prevention techniques, providing care and attention, and giving emotional support to the mother. The midwife received the wet little life into her gloved hands, tied and cut the cord, and then passed the crying naked newborn into the waiting naked hands of ... the cleaning lady! The bare-handed cleaning lady carried the newly born babe to the sink in the corner of the room, held him under the tap to wash off the blood, dried him off, wrapped him in a towel and handed him back to the midwife, who then handed the howling infant back to the mother.

'Wait a minute,' I said. 'What is all this about handing a newborn to the cleaning lady and her washing him under a sink? I thought we practised this in class! *You* are to dry and examine the baby, to make sure it's breathing, and to hand it immediately *to the mother* to maintain warmth, right?'

The Nepalese have a sweet way of bouncing their head from side to side, which can mean either 'yes' or 'no', depending on the situation. The midwife said to me, 'That is true' (bobbing head movement). 'However, neither I nor the mother belongs to the caste that touches blood on the newborn. If the mother touches him before he is cleaned, she will not only affect her karma, but that of her newborn son. The cleaning lady is the person who can touch the blood and clean off the baby for the mother.' My medical-model mind told me to insist on the Right Way to do things. My common sense and social-model self told me not to even attempt to change a 5000-year-old cultural value. So, we trained the cleaning lady in immediate newborn care, gave her gloves, and convinced her to clean off the blood with cloth and not water. And even though we had no scientific evidence to support this change in procedure, we did it because we are women with common sense who wanted healthy babies and mothers.

Midwives manage to make the essential connections, in terms of balancing technology with cultural values, and women's needs with well-intentioned interventions. This can point the way toward common-sense preventive measures and health policies that work. By understanding the existing competition inherent between the dominant bio-technological model and the traditional midwifery model of social-ecological-integrated care, university-educated midwives can work together with life-educated midwives to make essential connections with women and families to promote healthy pregnancies, childbirth and childrearing.

The more difficult issue might be the problem of connecting traditional midwives with the medical systems they need for emergency interventions. They can take part in training to recognise danger signs, intervene appropriately and transport to secondary or tertiary settings. This is a positive move, if the transport exists, if a hospital has trained personnel, correct medications or a blood bank, and other resources to intervene and save a life. Unfortunately, when the woman and her traditional midwife, who is the authority on birth and health in her community, arrive at the referral hospital, they enter another planet. Everyone from the receptionist to the surgeon is the authority on this planet. They often don't speak the same language as the midwife or the woman, don't know the cultural rituals, and sometimes don't really care. They want to save a life, 'deliver' a baby, and move on to the next patient. The midwives, nurses and doctors in Planet Hospital have the *authoritative knowledge* on health and illness care.

Definitions of authority

The term 'authoritative knowledge' (AK) has emerged from anthropological and sociological research. Robbie Davis-Floyd and Carolyn Sargent (1997) write in their book *Childbirth and Authoritative Knowledge* that AK is used to describe how a particular system of knowing exists among a group of peers, and that, by their consensus, it carries more weight than other systems of knowing. For example, master plumbers have more authoritative knowledge than apprentice plumbers. Editors have more than journalists, who have more than writing students. And, in her community, the traditional midwife has more authoritative knowledge than the mother giving birth. She even has more authoritative knowledge than the young university-graduated nurse or midwife in her village, because that university-trained 'professional' is an unknown entity among the traditional midwife's group of peers, which is her community. Authoritative knowledge is all about accountability in a community of practice – *not that the knowledge is correct, but that it counts* (Jordon 1992). Just as certain medical practices based on bad habits or fear may be incorrect, it still matters that other professional health providers believe those practices are correct.

A case in point is episiotomy. Millions of women around the world today receive this senseless surgical incision during childbirth upon the most tender and private part of their body. In Eastern or esoteric models, the perineum is seen as the basic first chakra. According to doctors and midwives trained in the medical model (their authoritative knowledge in their community of practice), the episiotomy has always been 'necessary'. Now, after 15 years and hundreds of scientific studies on thousands of women showing that 'necessity' to be false, in fact harmful, why do doctors and midwives continue this barbaric practice? Because again, authoritative knowledge is all about accountability in a community of practice – *not that the knowledge is correct, but that it counts.*

Anthropologists will tell us that this episiotomy ritual, or custom, is based on fears from medical anecdotes. The fear, generated by antique medical men not knowing women's anatomy, was based on the idea that the baby's head would 'get stuck' or that 'brain damage' may occur because of the force of the tiny cranium against the pelvis. In fact, the cranium of the baby, along with the force of uterine contractions, opens up the cervix (not the pelvis, a bony structure which is opened up by hormones during pregnancy) so the baby can be born. Birth had been accomplished this way for a hundred million years before doctors invented episiotomies. That cutting ritual occurred around the same time that the 'lying on your back to give birth' ritual occurred. Physically, it's almost impossible to push a baby out while flat on your back, so an episiotomy becomes necessary. Throughout history women have always given birth in the squatting position. But of course, the vertical position, a position where the woman is physically *above* the doctor, doesn't accommodate the doctor's demeanour or comfort.

As all home birth midwives know, childbirth can be a very sexual – even an orgasmic – experience for the physically, emotionally, or spiritually non-maimed woman. Yes, sexual and sensual. However, hospital births, which strip the woman of any dignity she may have felt before coming into that institution of illness care, illustrate another sad example of ritual based on AK. The whole point of most hospital rituals is to diminish a healthy woman to the role of patient, as opposed to a powerful giver of life. This makes her dependent on the authority figures, be it the nurse, the attendant with the wheelchair, the man at the gate with the keys, the midwife or the doctor. *They* are the ones with the authoritative knowledge in their community of practice. The pregnant woman and her partner just visit that community.

'Because birth is cultural and historical, it is also political, bound up with the exercise of power,' writes Ronald Grimes (2000) in his landmark book about ritual and life passages, *Deeply into the Bone*. Because of the politics and economics involved with birth, some voices are heeded while others are silenced or ignored. Because of fear-based beliefs from press, parents or peers, mothers and others become subjects of ritualised manipulation during pregnancy and childbirth. Loss of control and fear of chaos underlie countless hospital rituals.

In most cultures, we are taught from our first years to earn control and keep it: over our bowels and bladder, over our needs and wants, and later over events and our emotions. Think about how we raise little boys to control their emotions or how we train female medical students to value their intellect over their intuition. In nursing, midwifery and medical schools, we are taught to fear tradition and ritual from the unknown world of patients or, worse yet, the world of traditional healers. We separate the woman from her world, wheel her through the emergency room and welcome her into our own world of ritual.

During their antenatal visits, we teach pregnant women how to gain control over what we see as a potentially deadly, out-of-control situation. They are taught to 'Let the professionals take care of you . . . breathe in the Lamaze (or other name) method . . . pant and push when we tell you and how we instruct you . . . sit up/lie down/roll over/go to the bathroom/stay in bed . . . follow the rules and everything will turn out fine'.

Anthropologist Robbie Davis-Floyd (1992) argues that hospital procedures serve as rituals because they successfully fulfil important psychological needs.

- Individual needs of each staff person in the hospital for constant confirmation of the rightness of their technological interventions, and for ways to cope with something not really under their control, which threatens their technocratic model of birth.
- Individual needs of the woman giving birth for reassurance when faced with the unknown, for official recognition by society's designated authorities on birth, and for official confirmation of their belief systems.
- The important needs of the wider culture to ensure the effective socialisation of its citizens and thus society's perpetuation.

This last one has more of an impact than it may seem at first glance. How can simple hospital rituals assure socialisation of a citizen? Because vertical authority perpetuates hierarchies. Think about how rituals in any context promote and value conformity within a group. The whole point is control. Conformity helps everyone relax around an unknown factor, and it comforts them to count on a vertical line of authority. Congress members and conscripts are two examples. Membership rituals, years of university medical, nursing or midwifery school rituals, and hospital rituals that ensure dependency of the patient on the authority figure are other examples of how hospital procedures ensure the effective socialisation of its citizens and thus society's perpetuation based on an authoritative knowledge.

Using a wheelchair to mobilise a healthy pregnant woman is one example of a purpose-filled ritual. A pregnant woman demonstrates perfect ambulatory ability when she gets into a car/taxi/bus/donkey-cart or even walks and makes it to the hospital without a wheelchair. We must remember that hospital rituals help personnel reinforce their *assumption* that malfunction may occur at any time, that constant vigilance is necessary to intervene appropriately, and that everyone needs to believe in the medical model for it to work.

'To place a healthy woman in a wheelchair instead of allowing her to walk,' says Davis-Floyd, 'is to tell her that at the very least the hospital thinks of her as disabled and weak.' The first impression she makes on the staff, on her husband and on herself is one of passivity, of helplessness, of fragility. Her lower position encourages the nurses or doctors to talk down to her (literally) or to talk to the standing person at her side. She is seen, and encouraged to see herself, as someone who cannot walk, adding insult to injury, since walking during labour is one of the most beneficial things a woman can do to ease labour pains and promote regular contractions.

Other rituals like routine intravenous insertion, pitocin drips, fetal monitors, episiotomies, or any other common interventions, occur in hospitals all over the world to different degrees. But in almost every case the woman, who up until this moment may have trusted her body and trusted her partner to support her, must now transfer her trust to a complete stranger who may or may not be sympathetic to her wants and needs. This purpose-filled separation makes her even more dependent on the provider with his or her authoritative knowledge.

The translation of authoritative knowledge into policy

With the magic words *hospital policy*, two powerful messages appear. The first is that the hospital has the *right* to separate the woman from her trusted companion, thus holding higher authority than the family. The second is that the labouring woman belongs to the hospital institution and not to her family unit. It is hard to imagine a traditional midwife understanding or adhering to any of these rituals. Why would she? She knows that the mother is the authoritative person in the room giving life. The traditional midwife brings ritual to the birthing scene also, but her procedures are to adjust elemental forces around this woman and her baby to smooth the journey.

In antiquity and throughout the history of humanity, women stayed with a woman to help her go through her transformative process while giving birth, not only to bring into the world a new life form – *dar a luz* in Spanish means 'to give to the light' and signifies childbirth – but to give birth to her Self. A girl becomes a woman not just by menstruating, although that is an important life passage. A woman giving birth connects with all women throughout time. It is this connection that becomes our authority. And women don't have to give birth to understand the connectivity, compassion and creativity that accompany any of life's transformative processes. Growing through any creative or transformative process assures one's own authoritative knowledge, one's inner 'knowing'. The good news is that men can have this understanding and compassion as well. The bad news is that, stereotypically, men seek self-transformation through conflict (Hedges 2002).

This does not mean that men can only respond this way, though. Remember the old joke about choosing a male gynaecologist? 'Why would you go to a mechanic who never owned a car?' A very compassionate male obstetrician responded[1], 'I don't believe that genitals determine one's ability to relate, to connect, or to accompany. It has more to do with trusting the feminine side of ourselves'. The word midwife means 'with woman' and anyone who helps another person go through a life-transformative process, connecting to the endless flow of universal energy, remaining true to the feminine and nurturing sides of our selves, knows what it's like to midwife someone. Science shows us that childbirth becomes safer and easier when mothers are accompanied by other women, and particularly when one woman is dedicated to her. In most cultures that would be the traditional midwife. In modern cultures and in hospital settings, that person is usually not the nurse-midwife, the obstetric nurse or the doctor, but the doula.

The term 'doula', first suggested by anthropologist Dana Raphael (Kitzinger 1996), comes from Greek and refers to a woman who personally serves another woman. Based on their research, midwives Kroeger and Pascali-Bonaro (2004) conclude that 'continuous support by a lay woman during labour and delivery facilitates birth, enhances the mother's memory of the experience, strengthens mother–infant bonding, increases breastfeeding success, and significantly reduces many forms of medical intervention, including caesarean delivery and the use of analgesia, anaesthesia, vacuum extraction, and forceps'. Eleven other randomised controlled studies of women in public hospitals, a place where women normally receive no emotional support, reveal that 'companionship by another woman during labour results in mothers needing fewer pain medications, having fewer instrumental

---

[1] Personal correspondence with Dr Jeff Smith, ObGyn and adjunct professor at Johns Hopkins University in Baltimore, Maryland, 2004.

deliveries and less Caesarean sections. Babies arrive in better condition at birth, also' (Hodnett *et al.* 2007).

Of course, there is a place for intervention, antibiotics, surgery or rescue medicine when it is appropriate. The problem spirals into another kind of chaos when our society values one kind of authority *over* another, one kind of knowing *instead* of another, and interventions as a *substitute* for prevention. Indeed, some traditional rituals and practices may not be beneficial to the health of a pregnant, birthing, postpartum or lactating woman. Some rituals just help people to feel control over what seems to be a chaotic situation. We may learn to understand fear, discover from whence it comes, and understand how to work with it to get on the other side of it. That is another facet of growth and change where everyone wins.

Traditional midwifery, expert midwifery

Midwives around the world are inclined to emphasise relationship, links, correlation and connection. For example, a very interesting coalition arose in 2000 from a meeting in Ceará, Brazil, involving midwives and others from Mexico to Antarctica. This Latin American and Caribbean coalition has conferences, publishes articles, maintains websites, develops educational programmes, and conducts studies. They call themselves the *Red Latino Americano y Caribe para la Humanización del Parto y Nacimiento* (the Latin American and Caribbean Network for the Humanisation of Childbirth), known on their web page by the acronym RELACAHUPAN (www.relacahupan.com/menu.htm, accessed June, 2010) and they consist of more than 20 various national organisations. These organisations have petitioned for official recognition at the United Nations, the World Bank, the World Health Organization, the International Confederation of Midwives, and the United Nations Fund for Population Development. Among their members they have traditional midwives. They have just published a Declaration for the Practice of Traditional Midwifery in the Americas. Box 8.1 gives this in full.

Box 8.1   Relacahupan declaration for the practice of tradition-al midwifery in the americas

From: http://partera.com/pages_en/tpe.html

She is an independent essential and primary care provider during pregnancy, birth and postpartum and is recognized as such by her community and jurisdiction. She offers domiciliary services. She works in isolated communities in developing countries and sometimes she practices in developed

---

countries. She is a neighbor of the mothers she assists, and may be aboriginal in her country.

Her talents vary according to the region of residence. Her gift as a midwife and her intuition help create an intimate, unique relationship with each mother and infant under her care. The use of diets, plants, various infusions, immersion baths, sweat baths, incense, enemas and massages integrate her knowledge. She understands and uses minimal intervention and special maneuvers to work with the most difficult births. She practices hygiene, promotes breastfeeding, and protects the mother with her presence, advice and prayers. The traditional midwife considers birthing a natural event, for many it is a ceremony. The traditional midwife works and collaborates in the health of the newborn baby and takes care of her/him as long as is deemed necessary. She also takes care of the mother's health, offers education with regard to family planning and is accessible to help the women with her needs throughout her life.

She gets her knowledge from traditional, and informal methods ancient to the profession. This includes: learning through her own experience as a mother, assisting other women, from her ancestors, colleagues, healers, other health providers and by means of self-learning; dreams, examples from nature, spirits, her spirituality and God may guide her work. When her education comes from a non-governmental organization she is known as a trained traditional midwife. Occasionally she works in collaboration with other health providers. At times she may work in clinics and often she is the bridge between the health system and her community.

February, 2007

Case study – Guatemala

The city of Sololá hovers in green hillsides, 5 hours by bus from Guatemala City. Blooming, blood-red bougainvilleas drape pastel-colour stucco walls. Donkeys loaded with fresh vegetables clip-clop down cobblestone streets from the surrounding mountain communities and bring fresh food to town. The Guatemalan traditional midwives, termed *comadronas* in Spanish, live in the mountainous villages around Sololá and bring most of their neighbours into the world. They say they became midwives by happenstance because they have attended so many births, or because they felt chosen by God. They see themselves, and others in their community see them, as the cultural authority on pregnancy, labour, birth, postpartum and newborns.

Professional health providers in Sololá, graduates of medical and nursing schools, see themselves, and other professionals in the community see them, as the scientific authorities on pregnancy, labour, birth, postpartum and newborns. The public hospital in Sololá sits between tall eucalyptus trees on a flat piece of land just above the hilly town. The hospital offers 50 beds, along with an operating room, with two 'delivery' rooms. The administrator pulls nurses from other wards to attend a woman in labour because hospital births are such a rare event, whether that nurse is trained in obstetrics or not. In 1998, only 7% of babies in the entire province came into the world between elevated legs in cold steel stirrups on a gynaecological table under bright lights inside the Sololá Hospital.[2]

Guatemalan *comadronas* attend births at a woman's home the same way they have for centuries, with all the rituals and careful attention to details they learned from their mothers and grandmothers. *Comadronas* speak the same language as the mother (there are more than 150 native dialects in Guatemala). They spend more time with a mother at her home than a nurse can during a designated 8-hour shift at the hospital. *Comadronas* stay with the woman for days, nurture her with foods she likes to eat during labour and postpartum, give massages to alleviate labour pain, and perform precise rituals for the newborn that allow for a smooth transition from the spiritual world into its new earthly life. The obstetricians in Sololá never really accepted the idea of working with the *comadronas*. After all, they believed that traditional midwives were the cause of most maternal death and disease. There had been previous attempts to integrate *comadronas* into the healthcare system, but resistance to co-operation was high on both sides of the hospital door. Women didn't want to come into the hospital unless their *comadrona* came with them, and doctors would not accept *comadronas* or any other family members in the 'sterile delivery room'.

In 2005, Cornelia Muhl, a German midwife charged with training *comadronas* by her employer, Midwives for Midwives (a Guatemala non-governmental organisation)[3], did bring *comadronas* into the Sololá hospital, after extensive and exhausting personal meetings with doctors at the Ministry of Health in Guatemala City. Those physicians from the capital ended up *ordering* the obstetricians at Sololá to recognise a temporary truce and, for the sake of scientific study, accept some traditional midwives into the hospital for practical skills training … for 2 months.

Hired from Hamburg by Midwives for Midwives in Guatemala, graduated from a 5-year university midwifery programme with 5 more years of hospital practice, loaded with good Spanish language skills along with good intentions, Cornelia arrived in January from freezing Germany to tropical Guatemala. From February to April of 2005, she worked alongside 28 *comadronas* and four rural nurses in the Sololá hospital during nights, weekends, holidays, and any other time a labouring woman needed a midwife at her side for prenatal

---

[2] Personal correspondence, Dr Yadira de Cross, at that time a trainer of traditional midwives in Sololá and physician on staff at the hospital.

[3] womanway@aol.com and www.midwivesformidwives.com. For more information about the Midwives for Midwives organisation, visit www.midwifejennahouston.com/whoami.htm (accessed June, 2010).

care, childbirth, postpartum, newborn attention or family planning counselling. Cornelia used a training package with checklists and learning guides developed specifically for less literate *comadronas*[4], so she could objectively teach and measure the midwives' skills. These skills included taking blood pressure and vital signs, checking the position of the fetus with Leopold manoeuvres, timing the contractions using a watch with a second hand (most *comadronas* didn't have one or know how to use a watch), learning when a labour is prolonged and what to do if it is, massaging for pain reduction, resuscitating the adult and newborn, promoting breastfeeding immediately after birth, practising normal newborn care, and recognising postpartum haemorrhage, among other skills. It is important to note that *none* of these skills had ever been taught to *comadronas* in Guatemala before, even though they are the people who attend 90% of all births.

Nurses from the Ministry of Health government training programmes are instructed to teach traditional midwives how to mind their own business, to not replace the professionals, and to do only two things well: recognise danger signs and transfer. The nurses emphasise in the government training programmes that 'only professionally trained doctors and nurses' should care for a woman during her pregnancy and birth. This is not just a phenomenon of Guatemala or even Latin America, but worldwide. Cornelia, the German midwife, wrote in her Midwives for Midwives final report[5]: 'At first, the hospital personnel thought I must be a doctor training the midwives, even though I explained my degree and professional midwifery status. They couldn't imagine a midwife as a professional. I guess believing I was a physician made them feel better about my presence'. She also objectively and professionally noted which skills the *comadronas* and nurses learned well, and which ones they had difficulty with. She reported on the 11-week training results with German precision:

- We had 10 clinical days for each student, consisting of 7–8 hours a day, plus some overnight shifts of 12 hours, and some overtime when we had births. The average was 80–90 hours of clinical training per student.
- Each student had an average of three births: two as assistant and one as the principal midwife.
- Students attended 32 births, four of which were C-sections for failure to progress, defined by the doctor on duty.
- Students resuscitated (successfully) three babies. No babies died from our attendance.

---

[4] Developed by Metcalfe & Davenport/matronas, an independent consulting group to which the author belongs, and which wrote the guidelines according to WHO recommendations.

[5] The director of Midwives for Midwives, Jenn Houston, has the copy of the final report. She may be reached at www.midwifejennahouston.com/whoami.htm (accessed June, 2010).

- Students had one perineal tear (second degree), and students only had to cut one episiotomy.
- Of 111 prenatal appointments, each student had an average of five clients.
- Each student learned to do a complete clinical history and prenatal physical assessment, i.e. fundal heights measurements, fetal heart counting and listening, fetal position and presentation, vital signs, and counselling.
- Students gave postnatal care to 192 postpartum women, an average of 8–14 each.

It bears repeating that none of these skills or competencies had *ever* been taught to the traditional midwives before in any government-sponsored class. The midwives' tears of gratitude dampened their certificates during their graduation ceremony. Cornelia rarely showed emotion in her final report for Midwives for Midwives. In one instance she mentions that the students were very good about using the checklists, and they '. . . were very self-confident after the first month, and proud of themselves for the good job they did'. Only once did Cornelia offer an emotional yet diplomatic insight about staff relationships. She wrote, 'As we all know, to start working in the hospital was very hard. We encountered hostility with nurses and doctors every day. With time we started to make friends, and they started seeing us as helpers for their work. They did not give many prenatal appointments to us, but by the end they were giving us almost all their patients. With time we demonstrated that we were safe caregivers. They saw that we could resuscitate babies, that we were able to conduct births safely and with an intact perineum, that we could repair tears, that we could examine babies and help women to be safe and with good care. By the end they all knew that we used music, we allowed family to be with women, and that we used different positions for giving birth. In the last week they gave us two laboring women a day, maybe because they knew we were leaving'.

Cornelia and the other professional midwives working with Midwives for Midwives had much more to say personally about the treatment they and the mothers received in the hospital. They are horror stories, really, about doctors cursing *comadronas* in front of their clients, about professionals preferring to watch the finals of the regional football play-off on TV rather than attending the six women they had in labour, about losing blood samples, misplacing medications or not charting untoward events from their erroneous interventions, thus preventing subsequent investigation. These practices are not rare or even unusual. But it's also not hard to understand why doctors and nurses are territorial about their hospital rituals and practice. Their training, fears and habits guide them to want to control the outcome.

The Midwives' Association of North America (MANA), the International Association of Midwives (IAM)[6] and other organisations whose members

---

[6] See their websites for more information: www.mana.org/ and www.iam.org, and for more definitions see www.mana.org/definitions.html#MMOC (accessed June, 2010).

include Guatemalan *comadronas* recognise and respect traditional midwifery practices and also recognise that education and training are necessary during all our careers – be that traditional midwifery or university-graduated midwifery. They understand that women who value women for their creative powers are no threat to society: they are the reason that society survives. One of the most significant statements in the MANA list of midwifery values is the following:

> *We value our relationship to a process larger than ourselves, recognising that birth is something we can seek to learn from and know, but never control.*

Conclusion

One of the great controversies dividing pregnant women, midwives, physicians and Ministries of Health officials remains: do we train traditional midwives in life-saving skills, or not? Many studies have been done about this subject and others. Do we train more professionals and upgrade the hospital infrastructure? Why can't we do both? Who has the money for all this? What do we consider to be 'measurable outcomes' for all this intervention? Do we have the time to wait for midwifery students to graduate from a 4-year course and get out into the rural areas to see any results? Are formally trained midwives even accepted in rural areas by the people they serve? Most studies have shown that professional providers (midwives or doctors or nurses) *may* be accepted by the rural folk if and when they see immediate results that are beneficial to their physical health. But when it comes to spiritual and emotional health, the village midwife remains the best hedge against unforeseen circumstances, despite her lack of formal training.

Of course, government Ministries of Health in poorer countries don't agree. In a study from the University of Nairobi in Kenya (Kenya Ministry of Health 2003), the authors conclude that, 'Despite tremendous resources spent on them, the training of Traditional Birth Attendants[*] over the past two decades … has not reduced maternal mortality'. They credit any observed improvement after introducing TBA training programmes (government-dictated programmes, given by university-educated nurses) to the associated supervision and referral systems, or to the quality of essential obstetric services available at first referral level. First level means the health post. It could also mean the home, if the midwife was adequately trained in life-saving skills,

---

[*] Traditional birth attendants are otherwise known as 'TBAs', a deprecatory title used by most university-educated professionals for traditional midwives. These women call themselves midwives.

or if the mother, the midwife or the nurse had access to adequate supplies at the first-level referral center. This study (and many similar ones) mentions that a family's continued preference for traditional midwives is attributed to proximity to the woman's home, respectful attitude toward the mother and her family, and flexible modes of payment – things apparently lacking at the government health centre. The Kenya study also points out that distance and access to skilled attendance are factors that influence maternal deaths rates. How can the TBA resolve that problem? And how can any government dismiss the traditional midwife? As a respected South African literary magazine observes, traditional midwives have been an integral part of African medicine for centuries. This is not only because African people still love and fear the spirits, but also because a great number of the South African population do not have access to existing health services (Troskie 1997).

If you search Google for 'traditional midwife' you will find more than 861,000 entries. Much as they are ignored, deprecated, illegalised or trained to be something they are not, traditional midwives have always existed, since the beginning of time ... the world's oldest profession. Meanwhile, in Kenya, Guatemala, Indonesia, China, Paraguay, even the USA – wherever traditional midwives continue to serve women's and families' physical, spiritual and emotional needs in their communities – government doctors in charge of health policy for populations will continue to try to convince folks that they need to trust the institution of medical experts and all its technology. Curing and rescue interventions are quicker and easier than building health facilities, constructing the roads to reach them, equipping them, staffing them, training and paying staff, educating girls or eradicating poverty. Training traditional midwives to just recognise danger signs and transfer will not save more lives, because that philosophy disconnects the family, the decision makers in the community, and the spiritual, emotional or psychological components of pregnancy and childbirth. One way to incorporate traditional and other midwives into a medical model is to allow midwives to bring their clients into the hospital and stay with them. Then, the patient gets the best of both worlds: the midwifery model based on trust that birth works, and the medical model of care based on intervention in case of emergency.

Traditional midwives are not our little sisters, to be steered and brought around to our way of thinking. They are not misguided children who may someday learn to be like us adults. They do not practise witchcraft, voodoo or magic by trade, although they may incorporate aspects of that in their rituals. They may or may not have an art, a gift or a calling to practise midwifery. They do not know more than we do, either. They have some dangerous habits that need to be eliminated, just like we do. Some traditional midwives are illiterate, but that doesn't mean they are stupid. Some don't want to change, because it threatens them. Some want to learn new techniques in order to charge more for their services.

The majority of traditional midwives are called upon by the women and families they serve because they are trusted, whether or not they know what they are doing. And most of them do. Indeed, why would an underprepared and frightened fireman or policeman be trusted to attend a birth, when a well-prepared and confident traditional midwife is not? Expertise in midwifery involves science along with compassion, self-knowledge combined with people-skills, and it mostly involves trust: in the birth process, in the woman, and in ourselves. Traditional midwives know this. We can learn from their expertise and combine it with our own to make relationships stronger – which leads to healthier mothers, babies and families.

References

Andreason A (1995) *Marketing Social Change – Changing Behavior to Promote Health, Social Development, and the Environment*. Washington, DC, Jossey-Bass.

Davis-Floyd R (1992) *Birth as an American Rite of Passage*. Berkeley, CA, University of California Press.

Davis-Floyd R, Sargent C (eds) (1997) *Childbirth and Authoritative Knowledge – Cross Cultural Perspectives*. Berkeley, CA, University of California Press.

Gaskin I (1978) *Spiritual Midwifery*. Summertown, TN, The Farm Book Press.

Grimes R (2000) *Deeply Into the Bone – Re-inventing Rites Of Passage*. Berkeley, CA, University of California Press.

Hedges D (2002) *War is a Force That Gives Us Meaning*. New York, Anchor Books.

Hodnett ED, Gates S, Hofmeyr GJ, Sakala C (2007) Continuous support for women during childbirth. *Cochrane Database of Systematic Reviews* 3: CD003766.

Jordon B 1992 *Birth in Four Cultures: A Crosscultural Investigation of Childbirth in Yucatan, Holland, Sweden, and the United States*. Illinois, Waveland Press.

Kenya Ministry of Health, University of Nairobi, Population Council (2003) *The Kenya Safe Motherhood Demonstration Project*. Safe Motherhood Policy Alert, No.4. Nairobi, Kenya Ministry of Health.

Kitzinger S (1996) *The Complete Book of Pregnancy and Childbirth*. New York, Knopf.

Kroeger M, Pascali-Bonaro D (2004) Continuous female companionship during childbirth: a crucial resource in times of stress or calm. *Journal of Midwifery and Women's Health* 49(4)(suppl): 19–27.

Paluzzi J (2004) Primary health care since Alma Ata – lost in the Breton Woods? In Castro A, Singer M (eds) *Unhealthy Health Policy – A Critical Anthropological Examination*. New York, Altamira Press.

Richmond J (1990) Keynote address at the American Academy of Pediatrics Conference on Cross-national Comparisons of Child Health, Washington, DC, March.

Troskie TR (1997) The importance of traditional midwives in the delivery of health care in the Republic of South Africa. *Curationis* 20(1): 15–20.

Wagner M (1994) *Pursuing the Birth Machine – The Search for Appropriate Birth Technology*. Camperdown, Australia, ACE Graphics.

Part III
Collaboration

Introduction to Part III

Soo Downe

The three chapters in this section seek to unravel the meaning of collaboration, as opposed to teamworking or multidisciplinary practice. In the process, effective collaboration is viewed as a function of values and beliefs, and not simply a way of practising that is based on a specific set of tools or rules. The conclusion drawn is that working collaboratively calls for emotional intelligence, and for courage and determination, as the case studies in the section illustrate.

In Chapter 9, Soo Downe and Kenny Finlayson examine the etymology of the term 'collaboration'. They then unpick the differences between teamwork and collaboration, using Nicolescu's taxonomy of multidisciplinarity, interdisciplinarity and transdisciplinarity to move from a position where individuals occasionally cross clear boundaries to meet each other to one where roles, methods and viewpoints are combined and somewhat 'fuzzy'. The chapter goes on to examine a range of tools used to measure the nature and effectiveness of teamwork and collaboration, and to assess the utility of this work for maternity care. This leads in to an examination of the potential contribution of theories of boundary work, communities of practice, social networking and emotional intelligence, as routes to building understanding about how to develop and promote effective collaboration. The chapter concludes with the possibility that good collaboration practice might be an important route to working effectively within the complex system that is maternity care, to decrease toxic environments, and to increase salutogenic well-being for women and for staff.

Ngai Fen Cheung and Anita Fleming continue the values-based ethos of this section in Chapter 10. Using concepts of 'openness' and 'sharing', they present examples of effective collaboration in a range of settings. Anita presents specific examples of women with complex obstetric histories, who required care across traditional geographical, disciplinary and clinical boundaries. She demonstrates the skills and attitudes that are necessary to maximise women's choice and well-being in these circumstances. Fen takes a strategic line, describing the process she undertook to introduce the first birth centre ever set up in China. In both cases, it is evident that collaboration requires leadership, expertise, courage and a willingness to take calculated risks in pushing clinical, philosophical, personal and organisational boundaries.

Collaboration can also emerge unexpectedly from innovative initiatives. In Chapter 11, Alison Brodrick and her colleagues describe the process of developing a toolkit to reduce caesarean section. The work was set in motion by a UK Department of Health body, the Institute for Innovation and Improvement. They demonstrate the evolution of the toolkit as they began to engage with clinicians on the ground, and their realisation that building effective collaboration was central to its success. The quotes they provide from those engaging with the toolkit demonstrate that it has been catalytic in promoting important improvements in the quality of care in local sites. In a salutogenic analysis ('what works well'), the authors offer a list of characteristics for services that aspire to optimal care, based on the data emerging from their project. However, they also recognise the essential role of philosophy and belief in this success. As they say, 'Change can be driven and sustained through engaging with core values of individuals and mobilising their own internal energies and drivers for change ... In this way, shared understanding is promoted, leading to alteration in collective behaviours, and to collective action ...'.

To an extent, the chapters in this section demonstrate that collaboration requires mutual recognition of expertise, and the input of transformatory leaders, to be effective. The concluding pages in Chapter 12 bring these three aspects together into a synthesis that seeks to summarise the key messages of this book.

Chapter 9
Collaboration: Theories, Models and Maternity Care

Soo Downe and Kenny Finlayson

Introduction

The issue of collaboration is high on the healthcare agenda in many countries. It is perceived to be a risk management solution and a vector for maximising good-quality care. In the maternity services, collaboration is seen as particularly important for women who cross boundaries, from low- to high-risk status, or vice versa, or from one geographical place of birth to another. However, there has been very little discussion of the nature of collaboration or of the efficacy of various collaboration models. This chapter will examine a range of theories and models of collaboration. It will then examine collaboration in healthcare in general and in maternity care in particular. In the process, possible theories of collaboration are described and methods and approaches to measuring the effectiveness of these in healthcare practice are examined.

The nature of collaboration

Although the term 'collaborator' can have negative connotations, particularly in relation to collaborating with an enemy, its recent use in relation to business and healthcare has been generally positive:

> *to work jointly with others or together especially in an intellectual endeavour*[1]

[1] www.merriam-webster.com/dictionary/collaboration (accessed June, 2010).

Essential Midwifery Practice: Leadership, Expertise and Collaborative Working, first edition. Edited by Soo Downe, Sheena Byrom and Louise Simpson
Published 2011 by Blackwell Publishing Ltd.
© 2011 Blackwell Publishing Ltd.

and

> *the state of having shared interests or efforts (as in social or business matters)... the work and activity of a number of persons who individually contribute toward the efficiency of the whole.*[2]

The etymology of the word can be traced back to the Latin verb *collaborare*, which is a combination of 'together' (co-) and effort (-labor). This suggests that collaboration is a dynamic and active process between people that is generally directed towards doing and achieving something.

There does not appear to be any significant theoretical literature in the area of collaboration. Work that has been done on game theory, distributed cognition and co-operation versus competition is heavily directed at creating artificial intelligence systems that mimic human behaviour. Network theory, and some of the concepts underlying ideas of communities of practice, appear to provide a more relevant cognitive and behavioural basis for understanding human–human collaborative interactions. We will return to these ideas later in this chapter.

In the absence of a clear theoretical basis for the discussion of collaboration, it might be useful to focus on debates and studies that have examined the effects of working together in practice. This is less straightforward than it may appear to be as the words collaboration, co-ordination, co-operation and teamwork are often used interchangeably. It is not always clear if the subject under discussion is a group of people from one discipline where the composition is fairly fixed, a group from one discipline where membership changes frequently, a fixed group with cross-disciplinary membership or a wide-ranging group of staff who may work in a defined area or with a particular group of service users or customers, but who do not regularly meet together. This confusion indicates that there is more to collaboration than simply working together or being in the same physical space at the same time. In order to examine this in more detail, we turn to the definitions used, the processes that describe how people work together, the measures used to assess the outcomes of specific ways of working together and the outcomes identified by those measures.

Definitions

In an attempt to classify degrees of integration where activities lie across and between disciplines and groups, Nicolescu (2007) has defined three levels of so-called 'interdisciplinarity', with specific reference to

[2] www.merriam-webster.com/thesaurus/collaboration (accessed June, 2010).

research activities that cross perceived disciplinary boundaries. *Multi-disciplinary* relates to the study of one topic using standard methods from different disciplinary viewpoints. *Interdisciplinary* relates to the study of a topic where the methods and viewpoints of different groups are combined and *transdisciplinary* is 'what is between, across and beyond disciplines' (p.144).

Nicolescu is particularly interested in boundary work. He has defined disciplinary boundaries as:

> *the totality of the results – past present and future – obtained by the laws, norms, rules, and practises of a given discipline ... There are multidisci-plinary and interdisciplinary ... boundaries ... however, transdisciplinar-ity has no boundaries ....*

> (Nicolescu 2009, p.1)

Arguably, collaboration is about what happens when effective working takes place at boundary junctions between distinctly different groups. Nicolescu claims that individuals or groups can demonstrate a progression in terms of collaboration, termed the 'four practices' model. This starts with involvement, grows through achievability, moves on to the sharing of measures that help with goal attainment and, when successful, reaches the point where it fulfils the (deepest) motivations of the participants. This is seen as a spiritual journey as much as a chronological one. We return to the concepts of humanisation of care and of emotional intelligence as the basis for effective collaboration later in this chapter.

In a review of a specific set of nine research papers appearing in the *Journal of Applied Behavioral Science*, Wood and Gray (1991) make the claim that any effective definition of collaboration must address the question, *who is doing what, with what means, toward what ends?* Based on the data in the included papers, they conclude that:

> *Collaboration occurs when a group of autonomous stakeholders of a problem domain engage in an interactive process, using shared rules, norms, and structures, to act or decide on issues related to that domain.*

This is clearly more in the area of interdisciplinarity than transdisciplinarity, Indeed, Wood and Gray explicitly note that stakeholders must have some degree of autonomy or the result is a merger and not collaboration. A close reading of UK healthcare policy and strategy documents suggests that the area of most interest is interdisciplinary and interagency teamworking, as it is at boundary interfaces that the quality and safety of care are likely to be compromised. This is the territory illuminated by Wood and Gray. However, most work in the area of human co-operation and collaboration has been undertaken in the context of intra-team working (i.e. within the same discipline), as opposed to cross-boundary inter-team operations. The next section summarises some of the literature in the teamwork field.

Teamwork effectiveness

Studies of teamwork specifically, as opposed to more general systems of collaboration, tend to draw on change management theory, such as Herzberg's motivation-hygiene theory (Herzberg 1964) and Lewin's freeze phases (unfreeze, transition, refreeze; Lewin 1951). Various tools and programmes exist to measure and/or assess the processes of teamworking. These include Tuckman's four team development stages (forming, storming, norming, performing; Tuckman 2001). Studies that are focused on reaching an authoritative definition of teamwork tend to highlight structure as a valid measurement of effectiveness. In these instances, the number of team members and/or the personal characteristics of individuals within the team are related to theoretical models of teamworking. Belbin's 'team role descriptors' (2004) or derivatives of Jung's 'personality types' are often used in this way (Briggs & Myers 1980). Process measures have also been used.

By assessing the levels and quality of communication, decision making and participation in team member exchanges, researchers and organisational theorists aim to judge the operating effectiveness of teams. This is the approach used by Lemieux-Charles and McGuire (2006). According to these authors, organisational and contextual nuances may play a significant role in the success or failure of an intervention aimed at increasing team effectiveness. Intensive care unit teams, for example, work together for short periods of time under acute conditions in which team membership fluctuates regularly. Long-term palliative care teams, on the other hand, tend to be fairly stable, with team members working together over extended periods of time. An instrument developed in one or other of these environments may therefore be contextually sensitive. In addition, the structure of an organisation as well as the support offered to teams working within the organization may influence team effectiveness (Bower *et al*. 2003). By encouraging team autonomy and providing resources for training, senior management can foster a climate in which the potential for team effectiveness is enhanced (Weisman *et al*. 1993). With these organisational and contextual features in mind, Lemieux-Charles and McGuire (2006) outline a healthcare model, the Integrated Team Effectiveness Model (ITEM), which incorporates organisational context, task design, team processes, team psychosocial traits, and objective and subjective outcomes (Table 9.1).

Based on this synthesis, Lemieux-Charles and McGuire recommend that researchers need to develop models of effectiveness tailored to the

Table 9.1 Conceptual summary of ITEM scale (Lemieux-Charles & McGuire 2006).

Component	Impact (all positive unless otherwise indicated)
Context: organisational, cultural and structural	Primary care solo practice structure
	Adequacy of staffing and resources
	Ethic concordance between patients and staff
	Organisational culture that enhanced team orientation
	Patient-centred culture
	Negative: dispersion of services across several hospital/ healthcare settings
Task features	Higher caseloads with special groups (led to development of specialised skills)
	Rules and procedures
	Task clarity
	Clarity of leadership
	Clarity of goals
	Interdependence
	Quality improvement practices
Team composition	Not too large, not too small
	Trade-off between team satisfaction and quality of care
	Smaller teams positive for participation
	Varied by professional group or status
	Strongest among those with distinct focus to their work, lowest among those who were involved in other teams as well
	Professionals higher perception of team effectiveness than para-professionals
	Presence of team champion
	Willingness to learn
	Stability over time
	Those with greater autonomy
	Age and ethnic diversity
Team processes	Positive communication patterns
	Low levels of conflict
	High levels of collaboration, co-operation, participation, perceived influence
	Leadership
	Team climate (support for innovation, commitment to quality, clarity of objectives)
Team traits	Cohesion
	Shared norms

types of teams being studied, the relevant patient populations and care delivery settings, and the particular work processes operational in that setting. This has some resonance with the question we have discussed above: *who is doing what, with what means, toward what ends?*, posed by Wood and Gray (1991).

The relevance of organisational, contextual and personal factors for team effectiveness has been recognised by a range of disciplines.

Leggat (2007) examined the attitudes and approaches to teamworking of Australian health service managers. She found there was equal commitment to working collaboratively, to a quality outcome and to the organisation. She also found some gender-specific differences. Male managers used more transactional patterns, deriving their power from their position on the formal organisational structure. Women tended to use more transformational leadership techniques, and derived their power from personal characteristics. These leadership types are discussed in more detail in Chapter 1.

In the context of teamworking, these different approaches might have a powerful influence on team effectiveness. Indeed, in a recent ethnographic study of interprofessional interaction and negotiation among nurses, paramedical staff and medical staff in two general and internal medicine settings in Canada, Reeves and colleagues (2009) noted that interprofessional interactions were 'terse' with (largely male) medical interactions characterised by being unidirectional, and those of other (largely female) groups being richer and lengthier, and based on both clinical and social negotiations.

Studies taking a teamwork approach tend to be focused on stable, single-disciplinary groups and on the characteristics which render the group more or less efficient. This work is of relevance to stable healthcare teams. However, there is a particular issue for health and social care settings where collaborative boundary work is necessary to maximise the best care for service users.

Multidisciplinarity and interdisciplinarity in health and social care

Measuring collaboration

In a similar progressive framework to the 'four practices' model suggested by Nicolescu, the NHS Leadership Quality Framework (2006) proposes a hierarchy or maturity matrix of collaboration (Box 9.1). This taxonomy seems to be particularly focused beyond unidisciplinary teamworking and towards interdisciplinary cross-boundary activities. In a literature review of studies of interdisciplinary collaboration, sociologist Linda Bronstein (2003) identified a number of factors that constitute the nature of collaboration, as well as several factors which influence collaboration in practice. She then used these to develop a tool to measure collaboration within the social work field. Features like interdependence, shared ownership of goals and flexibility are encompassed in many of the 42 questions used in the instrument. Several influencing factors, including structural (organisational) characteristics,

---

Box 9.1 NHS leadership qualities framework: collaborative working (NHS 2006)

0 Goes it alone
- Fails to involve others in bringing about integrated healthcare.
- Does not share information with other stakeholders.

1 Appreciates others' views
- Expresses positive expectations of internal and external stakeholders.
- Acknowledges and respects others' diverse perspectives.

2 Works for shared understanding
- Shares information with partners when appropriate.
- Summarises progress, taking account of differing viewpoints, so as to clarify understanding and establish common ground.
- Surfaces conflict and supports resolution of this conflict.

3 Forges partnerships for the long term
- Maintains positive expectations of other stakeholders, even when provoked, and strives to create the conditions for successful partnership working in the long term.
- Is informed on the current priorities of partners, and responds appropriately to changes in their status or circumstances.
- Ensures that the strategy for health improvement is developed in a cohesive and 'joined-up' manner.

---

a past history of effective collaboration and personal characteristics, are also incorporated.

In a subsequent review of instruments designed to measure nurse–physician collaboration, Dougherty and Larson (2005) identified five pertinent questionnaires. All of them used Likert-type scales to measure perceptions of collaboration, and most were developed and/or validated in an ICU environment. The oldest of these instruments (Weiss & Davis 1985) adopts a relatively simple ten-question strategy utilising two separate measurements: an assertiveness scale for nurses and a collaborative scale for physicians. This is an interesting reversal of the classic healthcare hierarchy where nurses are held to have little power and doctors are deemed to be dictatorial (Dougherty & Larson 2005). The tool is explicitly designed to challenge this hierarchy. This may limit its applicability as it does not acknowledge that health systems are more nuanced than the classic stereotypes suggest. Contemporary derivatives of this original Weiss and Davis format incorporate more comprehensive and finely tuned interpretations of collaboration. The Jefferson Scale of Attitudes toward Physician–Nurse Collaboration, for example (Hojat *et al.* 1999), monitors nurse–physician attitudes towards authority, autonomy, responsibility, shared decision making, role expectations and collaborative education.

Promoting collaboration

Most of the published accounts of interventions designed to promote interdisciplinary working are US-based evaluations of educational techniques. Buck and colleagues (1999) designed an interdisciplinary core curriculum that included staff from the areas of nursing, health science, physical therapy, dental hygiene, medical technology, radiological sciences and respiratory therapy. The Downstate Team-Building Initiative (DTBI) engaged with students from a range of health professions (Hope *et al.* 2005), and Swanson *et al.* (1998) report on a specific initiative at the University of Iowa known as the Integrated Health Professions Program. Horak *et al.* (2004) describe a multimethod approach to team building between nurses and physicians. This included a sensitivity session, coaching with nursing managers and ground rules for nurse and physician collaboration. The study took an appreciative approach, looking for what each group valued in the other group members, and what each could do for the other. There were clear positive changes in attitude, communication, patient care and morale, and these were reported by staff in both groups.

In contrast, the introduction of the Medteams training programme to staff of a range of professions and grades in seven labour and delivery wards in the United States (Harris *et al.* 2006) had mixed success. The programme involved translation of the principles of effective team behaviours from the aviation industry into healthcare, with the intention of improving safety. While there were some benefits to the project, the authors noted that simply forming teams without paying attention to local cultures and norms, and without getting buy-in from staff at all levels, limited the potential success of the programme.

Three Cochrane reviews have addressed this topic. Zwarenstein and Bryant (2000) examined interventions to promote collaboration between nurses and doctors. They located two trials, involving 1945 people. One evaluated daily, structured, multidisciplinary ward rounds that included nurses, doctors and other professionals in joint decision making. The other assessed the impact of a multidisciplinary ward round conducted four times a week. The reviewers conclude that these kinds of ward rounds made moderate improvements in length of stay and hospital costs. Significantly, they also note that such studies present complex logistical challenges, and that qualitative research should be undertaken to understand the basis on which future trials in this area should be performed. Given the general lack of a coherent theoretical underpinning for collaboration, this challenge might be met by paying attention to the suggested processes for the evaluation of complex interventions, proposed by the Medical Research Council (2008).

In the second relevant Cochrane review, Reeves and colleagues assess the impact of interprofessional education (IPE) on disparate staff groups (Reeves *et al.* 2008). Interprofessional learning at undergraduate and continuing education levels has been widely proposed as a mechanism for promoting mutual understanding and collaborative working. Reeves and colleagues located six studies in this area. Across four of these studies, IPE had a positive impact on emergency department culture and patient satisfaction; collaborative team behaviour and reduction of clinical error rates for emergency department teams; management of care delivered to domestic violence victims; and mental health practitioner competencies related to the delivery of patient care. Two reported both positive and neutral results. However, the authors note that all the studies were small and heterogeneous, and that they displayed methodological limitations. They conclude that it is therefore not possible to draw generalisible inferences from the data presented.

In the third review, Zwarenstein and colleagues examined the effect of collaborative practice-based interventions on professional practice and healthcare outcomes (Zwarenstein *et al.* 2009). In the five studies included, collaboration was operationalised through interprofessional rounds, interprofessional meetings or externally facilitated interprofessional audit. The authors conclude that there was some evidence for benefit of this kind of intervention but, again, that the available studies were too small and too heterogeneous to be entirely convincing. As before, the authors call for better theorising through qualitative research, and for trial designs that pay attention to context and complexity, such as cluster randomised trials.

Collaboration in the maternity care context

The current situation

There is clearly a problem with maternity care outcomes across the world. Despite the enormous health gains that have been generated by improving social circumstances and by the application of increased knowledge about human biophysiology, the one Millennium Development Goal that is not improving is the one that relates to maternal health and, specifically, maternal mortality. At the same time, rates of routine intervention for healthy women and babies in normal childbirth have reached epidemic proportions in both resource-rich and resource-poor countries. This is not a benign occurrence. Recent studies have indicated that, above a certain level, high rates of intervention may be harmful for both women and babies (Declercq *et al.* 2007; Kilsztajn *et al.* 2007; MacDorman *et al.* 2008).

The inverse care law, brought to general attention by the Black Report 30 years ago (Black 1980), is still operational in maternity care as in other areas of social life. As an example, in low-resource countries, women with higher socio-economic status tend to have excessive levels of caesarean section, while those of low socio-economic status have excessively low rates of childbirth interventions (Belizán *et al.* 1999). For both groups of women and babies, this imbalance carries iatrogenic risks.

A reading of the general maternity care literature suggests that influential childbirth analysts from a range of disciplines, including midwives, anthropologists, sociologists and feminists, seem to have reached a common conclusion on the history of maternity care and on its current state in a modernist world. That is, those in power dictate social (and thus maternity care) norms. Those in power are men, so these norms are patriarchal and masculinist (Arms 1975; Donnison 1977; Oakley 1985; Martin 1987). Since the powerful players in healthcare are physicians, the norms for healthcare are biomedical (Arney 1982). Obstetricians are generally male and hold power, so maternity care is based on masculinist, biomedical norms.

It appears that this philosophy has been readily adopted by authoritative midwifery authors and leaders across the world to the point that the term 'medicalisation of childbirth' is taken for granted as a description of modern maternity care which does not need to be challenged or problematised. In this climate, it is a short step to making the assumption that the overtreatment of many women in childbirth is due to (risk-averse) medicalisation, while the undertreatment of others is due to the excessive concentration of resources in centralised hospitals, resulting in the deaths of relatively impoverished women who cannot or will not access these centres of excellence.

The problem with these kinds of assumptions is that they result in a polarised blame culture. Doctors claim that midwives wilfully deny women pain relief for labour or refuse to accelerate normal labour artificially, based on professional self-interest and outdated ideals of the natural and the normal. These claims are based on the apparently obvious benefits of a short, pain-free labour. Midwives blame obstetricians for excessive intervention of childbirth, based on the assumption that this is a way of exercising the medical power base and of keeping women within obstetric control. Neither group seems to acknowledge that the choices women make may be heavily influenced by both midwifery and obstetric professional projects, by social pressures and by a general lack of trust in caregivers. In the service of their respective causes, there are some indications that women may be commandeered into one camp or the other. Annandale (1987) demonstrated this process in terms of midwife-led birth centres in her ethnography of a birth centre in the UK where women who chose to book with the birth centre became highly allegiant to the philosophy and beliefs of the birth centre midwives, sometimes in opposition to the views and attitudes of friends and family.

On the other side of the equation, as Denis Walsh has noted in Chapter 7, Machin and Scamell (1997) observed what they termed the 'irresistible biomedical metaphor' at work in centralised hospitals. In their study, women who attended NCT classes and who, therefore, may be assumed to be interested in normal childbirth were assimilated into the use of intervention once they entered the centralised hospital for birth.

All of this results in a polarised culture of maternity care where both professional groups operate on the basis that the other group is putting its own professional interests before those of childbearing women and their babies. There are many individuals who are genuinely dedicated to doing the best for the women and babies in their care, but there is good evidence that this authentic concern might be overwhelmed by the powerful oppositional forces that operate in many maternity care settings, as illustrated by the studies referred to above.

In a fascinating study of nurse-midwives and obstetricians, Simpson *et al.* (2006) examined this area of professional interaction. The research was undertaken in four US hospitals, each of which had between 3000 and 6000 births a year, and all of which had a predominantly nurse-midwife managed model of care. Fifty-four nurses were interviewed in eight focus groups and 34 obstetricians were interviewed individually. Two clear clinical areas of contention emerged: the use of routine fetal monitoring and the administration of pitocin or 'pit' (artificial oxytocin) for the induction and/or augmentation of labour. Accounts from the nurse-midwives revealed both clinical and interpersonal issues relating to these areas.

> *They [the physicians] like that pit pushed and you'd better push it and go, go, go, otherwise they'll be hot, really mad if it's not going.*

> *I would be petrified if at 7 am they* [the physicians] *walked in and I didn't have the pit going. They'd yell at me and that's just an added stress.*

This study provides some fascinating insights into the way both groups think and it includes a section that illustrates the problem of people exchanging information but failing to communicate.

> Nurse-midwife: *If I really think she* [the patient] *needs a section and I want them* [the physician] *to come over, I use key words … 'going no*

where, head is sky high, she's stuck, not changing even with good contractions'.

Obstetrician: *When I'm busy in the office or in the middle of the night, I'm listening for key words or phrases that mean I have to come . . . like fetal distress, lots of blood, prolapsed cord, ready for delivery . . . otherwise I know they don't need me right away. I can't come in for every call.*

In this example, both sides think they have a shared understanding of which words should trigger attendance at an emergency, but they are listening for different words. The careful use of specific linguistic cues (even if they are not actually successful) suggests a lack of trust and mutual respect between the two groups. It does not seem to be possible for doctors and midwives to trust each other enough for the nurse-midwives simply to say, 'this is an emergency, please come', and for the doctor to believe them and to come. These subtle linguistic rules present a significant risk to the mother and baby when they are not coded in the same way by doctors and midwives, as appears to be the case in this study.

Possibly surprisingly, it was some of the obstetricians who felt most hard done by in this situation, as they struggled to occupy territory that was fiercely guarded by the nurse-midwives.

Sometimes I feel downright unwelcome when I show up on the unit to check my patient without being called. The nurses say . . . 'What are you doing here? I didn't call you'.

As the authors conclude, 'Nurses and physicians shared the common goal of a healthy mother and baby but did not always agree on methods to achieve that goal . . .'.

This situation is mirrored by a paper reporting on the views of junior doctors working in maternity care in the north east of England (Pinki *et al.* 2007). The doctors were sent a survey asking them about collaboration issues with midwives. While the majority of the 68 who responded were positive about these relationships, a significant minority were not. Nearly a quarter of respondents (22%) reported midwives to be disrespectful and argumentative. More than two-thirds (69%) reported that they did not get a chance to examine women on the labour wards because of the midwives. Half (53%) felt that there were communication issues between junior doctors and midwives that needed to be addressed. There was no parallel survey of midwives, so these accounts are only from one particular viewpoint. An earlier study from Australia suggests that part of the issue might be dissonance between what midwife mentors thought junior doctors should learn, and the activities the doctors themselves believed they should be involved in

(Quinlivan *et al.* 2003). This kind of finding at the level of junior doctors suggests that opposition between midwives and medical staff might be set up at an early point for career obstetricians. If the findings are generalisible, this early antagonism might follow through when the juniors become more senior, setting up a self-perpetuating pattern between midwives and doctors that is echoed at all levels of the organisation (a 'fractal' structure in complexity theory terms). As doctors move regularly, this antagonism may also become viral, resulting in a widespread expectation that collaboration is likely to be difficult. Similar findings in a recent study undertaken in Australia suggest that the problem is widespread, and persistent (Reiger & Lane 2009).

Collaboration in maternity care strategy and policy: UK context

Over the last 10 years the UK government's agenda for health has aimed 'to develop a patient-led NHS that uses available resources as effectively and fairly as possible to promote health, reduce health inequalities and deliver the best and safest healthcare' (DH 2006a, p.5). In order to fulfil the requirements of this approach, many policies have been directed towards patients and, in particular, patient choice (DH 2000). Within maternity care, initiatives designed to expand and enhance the child-bearing experience encompass most aspects of provision, from antenatal care and birth to postnatal care (DH 2004, 2007).

With regard to place of birth, the Maternity Matters 'national choice guarantees' (DH 2007, p.5) state that women should be given three options: home birth (supported by a midwife), hospital birth (supported by obstetricians, midwives and anaesthetists) or birth in a midwife-led unit (supported by midwives). Whilst the vast majority of UK babies continue to be born in hospital, evidence from the National Childbirth Trust (2004) suggests that up to 75% of low-risk women might prefer to give birth in smaller, midwife-led units (MLUs), if they were available. At present not all regions of the UK have MLUs (either freestanding or adjoining the local hospital) although the intention was to have these facilities universally available by 2009 (DH 2007). As far as home births are concerned, recent figures would suggest that this option is being adopted by a small but increasing number of women (Redshaw *et al.* 2007).

From a provider perspective, the continued expansion and diversification of maternity services require careful planning, especially in areas where safety may be of concern. Given the increased emphasis on community-based approaches to antenatal care and the increasing numbers of women who wish to give birth in MLUs or at home, there are obvious safety implications for women who develop pregnancy complications antenatally or during labour. Although well-defined procedures currently exist for the transfer of complicated pregnancies from midwife-led care to obstetrician-led care (NICE 2007), anecdotal evidence suggests that both the effectiveness of these procedures and women's views of the transfer process are highly dependent on the quality of communication between health professionals.

The frequency of transfer varies widely both within and across regions, but studies would suggest that complications identified between the initial antenatal booking appointment and labour lead to the transfer of between 29% and 67% of women from midwifery-led care in hospital-based birth centres to obstetrician-led care in the local obstetric unit (Hodnett *et al.* 2005). Formal evidence equating the quality of midwife–obstetrician communication during the transfer of care with adverse perinatal outcomes is limited, but data from CEMACH (Confidential Enquiry into Maternal and Child Health) suggest that substandard levels of interprofessional communication can and do affect maternal outcomes, including maternal mortality (Lewis 2007).

This reinforces a theme in the previous CEMACH report which found that 'lack of communication and teamwork both within obstetric and midwifery teams and in multidisciplinary teamworking' contributed to the deaths of a number of women (Lewis 2004, p.7). The report goes on to highlight specific areas of weakness, notably at the initial booking visit and while arranging the transfer of women. It is during these situations that crucial clinical information may not be passed on to relevant professionals, and the potential for substandard care is increased. This may be confounded by disagreement between individuals and professional groups as to when booking should be in central units or when transfer should take place. High levels of interprofessional collaboration (including GPs, social workers, community mental health teams, accident and emergency staff as well as obstetricians and midwives) are recommended around booking and transfer with an emphasis on standardising guidelines and protocols (Lewis 2004).

For many years, teamwork was promoted as an ideal approach to optimising care delivery. As we have mentioned, the effectiveness of this system of staff organisation is complicated by the fact that the day-to-day working of most maternity care teams (interpreted as a group of people who are all at work in the same geographical space and over the same period of time, providing care for a defined group of women, such as all those labouring in one labour ward over one defined period) rarely involves the same midwives, obstetricians, anaesthetist, paediatrician, healthcare workers, nurses, reception staff, doulas, and so on from one day to the next. The elements of the 'team' in this context are not fixed, and are constantly shifting.

In addition, particularly in maternity care, previous strategic moves towards teamworking have been translated into the creation of loosely affiliated hierarchical groups where the final decision on policy and practice is made by those at the top of the hierarchy (usually senior obstetricians). This interpretation of teams was operationalised by protocols and procedures that were nominally agreed by the 'team' but which were usually designed and signed off by a powerful minority of representatives of the key disciplines involved. The 'teamness' was then measured by how well the group as a whole adhered to these agreed approaches to care.

This history has tended to create resistance to teamworking as a concept in UK maternity care. Indeed, there is evidence that even where groups are nominally working as teams, ineffective care can arise. In the UK, the example of Northwick Park Hospital serves to illustrate the point. Northwick Park has elevated rates of high-risk pregnancy and birth. However, even given this caseload, the incidence of maternal mortality reported by the hospital between 2002 and 2005 seemed to be higher than expected. As a consequence, the national Health Care Commission undertook an in-depth review of maternal mortality at the hospital (Health Care Commission 2006). They found that the rate was indeed much higher than expected and concluded that a number of issues underpinned this problem, including systems for risk management and lack of clinical leadership. One of the most important issues identified was poor inter- and intraprofessional relationships between midwives and consultant obstetricians. It seemed that being in a nominal 'team' was not enough. In the same year as this report was published, the Department of Health produced a document entitled *In the Patient's Interest: Multi-professional Working Across Organisational Boundaries* (DH 2006b). In this paper, the government talked about both collaboration and teamwork as separate but interlinked entities. However, 2 years later, the King's Fund report on safety in maternity care (King's Fund 2008) devoted a whole chapter to the importance of teamworking in maternity care as a fundamental component of a safe system, but made very little mention of collaboration.

As illustrated by these policy-level documents, there is little dispute about the value of working across boundaries in healthcare in general, and in maternity care in particular. However, as we have also indicated, it is far less apparent that healthcare systems can measure or create collaboration because authoritative, universally acceptable methods of doing this have not yet been developed.

Considerations for a theory of interdisciplinary collaboration

As we have noted, collaboration is a complex, nuanced and multifaceted issue. Research studies undertaken in this area suggest that several key factors are likely to be relevant in the development of collaborative working (in its broadest sense). These include:

- clear and respected boundaries
- conflict resolution
- participation and cohesion
- shared mental models including mindful interdependence (Lyndon 2006)
- open and honest communication
- mutual trust
- interdependence
- shared responsibilities.

Given that interdisciplinary working is the area of primary interest in maternity care, in this section we raise and briefly discuss three possible areas for future philosophical and theoretical debate and investigation in this specific domain of collaboration. The first is the contribution of boundary work, social network theory and communities of practice. The second is the role of emotional intelligence. The third is the potential for complexity and salutogenesis to act as a framework for analysing the important components of effective collaborative in practice.

The contribution of boundary work, communities of practice and social network theory

In a recent review of approaches to evaluating the success of interdisciplinary and transdisciplinary research, Klein (2008) proposes seven generic principles for effective inter- and transdisciplinary working in research: variability of goals; variability of criteria and indicators; leveraging of integration; interaction of social and cognitive factors in collaboration; management, leadership and coaching; iteration in a comprehensive and transparent system; and effectiveness and impact.

For a number of these principles to be operationalised, effective working across disciplinary boundaries is essential. Boundary work theory originated as an analysis of the division between science and non-science (Gieryn 1983). More recently, it has come to refer to any academic/scientific situation in which demarcations between academic disciplines collide, creating the need to defend domains as belonging to one discipline or another. The fact that these kinds of debates can take place indicates the socially constructed nature of such boundaries.

Gieryn defined boundary work as the 'attribution of selected characteristics to [an institution] (i.e. to its practitioners, methods, stock of knowledge, values and work organization) for purposes of constructing a social boundary that distinguishes some intellectual activities as [outside that boundary]'. If the term 'intellectual activities' is replaced with 'clinical practices', the definition could apply equally well to healthcare professionals as to academic disciplines.

In a further development of the theory, the idea of 'boundary objects' has been developed (Star & Griesemer 1989). These refer to abstract or actual elements that transcend disciplinary boundaries, therefore, in principal, improving the potential for collaboration. One such 'object' could be communities of practice or CoPs (Wenger *et al.* 2002). Wenger and colleagues note that:

> *crossing boundaries requires building trust not only inside communities, but through sustained boundary interactions ... we would even argue that the learning potential of an organisation lies in this balancing act between well developed communities and active boundary management.*

> (p.154)

They argue that CoPs can be formed both within so-called 'sticky' boundaries (where groups are internally cohesive and there is little transfer externally) and across 'leaky' boundaries, where knowledge and interaction can flow freely. It could be hypothesised that, in many settings, professional groups in maternity care have highly sticky boundaries, as exemplified by the stereotypical views of each other noted above. This would also explain why working in 'teams' in the same geographical space doesn't of itself lead to effective collaboration. Sticky boundaries are particularly likely to block Klein's fourth principle – interaction of social and cognitive factors in collaboration. The creation of CoPs as boundary objects might allow for increased boundary permeability and, therefore, increased collaboration.

Such initiatives would need to be instituted with caution. One of the principles of CoPs is that they cannot be effective if they are artificially created. They are emergent phenomena. As Wenger (1998) has said:

> *... what makes it a community – is its practice ... Such a concept of practice includes both the explicit and the tacit ... what is said and what is left unsaid; ... the implicit relations, the tacit conventions, the subtle cues, the untold rules of thumb, the recognizable intuitions, the specific perceptions, the well-tuned sensitivities, the embodied understandings, the underlying assumptions, the shared worldviews, which may never be articulated, though they are unmistakable signs of membership in communities of practice ...*

> (p.47)

This raises the question of how a CoP occurs if boundaries are very sticky, and they can't be constructed artificially. Social network theory may provide a solution. Social networks map the relationships between 'nodes' (individuals, organisations, groups), paying attention to the existence and strength or weakness of the 'ties' between the nodes. These ties denote the relationships between each nodal point in the network. The relationships can be expressed graphically. These network maps delineate tightly or loosely connected groups. They can also demonstrate which individuals in the network cross boundaries, by having ties both in and between tightly networked groups. It is these individuals who are most likely to be catalytic in forming CoPs.

The role of emotional intelligence

As has been noted in Chapter 1, 5 and 6, emotional intelligence appears to be a key component of effective transformational leadership and of adaptive, or integrated, expertise. Given the affective elements of collaboration that have arisen in some of the research discussed above, it is possible that any attempt to catalyse effective collaboration will need to capitalise on group members who are highly emotionally effective. For the purpose of our argument in this section, we combine the definitions of Salovey and Mayer (1990), who understand emotional intelligence to be a combination of emotional perception, emotion use, understanding of emotion and emotion management, with that of Bar-On (2006), who defines emotional intelligence as being concerned with effectively understanding oneself and others, relating well to people and adapting to and coping with the immediate surroundings in order to be more successful in dealing with environmental demands.

Goleman (1995), who popularised the concept of emotional intelligence, has said:

> *Emotional intelligence* [is] *self-awareness, altruism, personal motivation, empathy, and the ability to love and be loved by friends, partners, and family members. People who possess high emotional intelligence are the people who truly succeed in work as well as play, building flourishing careers and lasting, meaningful relationships ...*

People who are highly networked, and who demonstrate both central and distributed ties on social network diagrams, are likely to be emotionally intelligent. Hunter (2004) suggests that emotion work with colleagues can be one of the most challenging aspects of maternity care and, given the results of the studies of Simpson *et al.* (2006) and Pinki *et al.* (2007) described above, it is likely that collaborative initiatives will need to pay close attention to emotionally intelligent individuals, and to their capacity to catalyse positive change.

Complexity and salutogenesis as a framework

As maternity care and interdisciplinary working are complex by nature, it is unlikely that simple models of maternity care collaboration will have high explanatory power. Even if the need to look for complexity is acknowledged, studies of systems that have gone wrong, like Northwick Park, will only reveal the problem. To find solutions, it is important to look at how complex systems succeed – to examine settings where collaboration is evident and effective despite the barriers of public healthcare systems. One of us has previously argued for the need for a salutogenic ('generation of well-being') stance to understand maternity care systems (Downe & McCourt 2008). From this perspective, we are interested in what makes things go right, as well as what might make them go wrong. In addition, following complexity theory approaches, we take the view that health systems are not simple and linear but complex and interconnected. Under this hypothesis, organisations are fractal, as noted above (Downe 2010). The attitudes, approaches, beliefs and practices tend to be 'self-similar' between one level of the organisation and another. As all the levels are strongly interconnected, small changes at one level can also resonate strongly across all levels, and this provides opportunities for rapid, often unexpected change.

For example, one birth experienced positively can make all those who were involved feel joyful and fulfilled. The sense of well-being that this engenders can be transmitted through telling the story of the event to others who were not there. This creates positive energy and a virtuous cycle that stands in opposition to vicious circles of mutual misunderstanding, distrust and increasing polarisation, characteristic of non-collaborative settings. It is also true that in highly connected fractal systems one negative event, like a litigation case, can send the system spiralling downwards if it has very sticky boundaries which restrict the opportunity to see a wider picture. Those experiencing negative events within sticky boundaries cannot benefit from cross-boundary supportive discussion and debate that would make the event an opportunity to learn and develop for the future. As Kelly and Allison (1998) have noted, in terms of complex adaptive organisations:

> *Before it can be effective, an organisation must dismantle its vicious cycles . . .*

> (p.63)

> *Decisions made in ignorance backfire, leading to mistrust. People learn not to entrust their individual survival to others in the group. Mistrust amplifies the fear and the cycle intensifies . . .*

> (p.54)

The major hurdle is to remove the underlying fear of telling the truth ...

(p.56)

Each person must become a fully responsible autonomous agent who respects the rights of others to assume similar status.

(p.66)

Having reached the theoretical conclusions set out in this chapter, we came across a recent paper that has brought together some of the insights from boundary work theory, network theory and complex adaptive systems to propose an approach that might maximise safety in healthcare (Braithwaite *et al.* 2009). The authors undertook a wide-ranging review of literature from mathematics, sociology, marketing science and psychology. They conclude that progress in terms of organisational safety 'involves the use of natural networks and exploiting features such as their scale-free and small world nature, as well as characteristics of group dynamics like natural appeal (stickiness) and propagation (tipping points)'.

They recognise the need to build on what is important to local staff, to work with local expertise in natural groups based on interests and preferences (as in classic community of practice theory) and on naturally occurring characteristics of complex systems. The approach they recommend includes nurturing aspects which chime with emotionally intelligent approaches. It appears that current analysis in the field of collaboration is moving towards a more theoretical, integrated approach.

Conclusion

In this chapter, we suggest a way of moving towards an understanding of collaboration which acknowledges that all labours and births are unique, and that all are based on a complex and delicate synergy between mother and baby, mother, baby and partner, and mother, baby, partner and caregivers, as well as many other interconnected influences. In this mix, the connectivity between midwife and obstetrician is an important element. In the absence of a general theory of collaboration, we propose that future studies in this area need to pay attention to the inter-relationship of the history of the groups who need to collaborate, the context in which they are operating, their personal characteristics, and their beliefs and values related to the area in which the collaboration is needed. Reference to boundary and emotion work theories, to the nature of the local social networks and to the role of emotional intelligence might provide a useful framework for creating change in the future. This process could be maximised if maternity care provision is recognised to be a complex adaptive system in the local context and if attention is paid to places where collaboration is working well, despite the apparent presence of barriers and confounders. Communities of practice might be a powerful force for change if they are allowed to emerge spontaneously and to evolve naturally over time.

References

Annandale EC (1987) Dimensions of patient control in a free–standing birth center *Social Science and Medicine* 25(11): 1235–48.

Arms S (1975) *Immaculate Deception: A New Look t Women and Childbirth in America*. New York, Bantam Books.

Arney WR (1982) *Power and the Provision of Obstetrics*. London, University of Chicago Press.

Bar-On R (2006)The Bar-On model of emotional–social intelligence (ESI). Psicothema 18(suppl): 13–25.

Belbin RM (2004) *Management Teams: Why They Succeed or Fail*, 2nd edn.Oxford, Butterworth Heinemann.

Belizán J, Althabe F, Barros FC, Alexander S (1999) Rates and implications of caesarean sections in Latin America: ecological study. *British Medical Journal* 319: 1397–402.

Black N (1980) *Black Report. Inequalities in Health: Report of a Research Working Group*. London, Department of Health and Social Security.

Bower P, Campbell S, Bojke C, Sibbald B (2003) Team structure, team climate and the quality of care in primary care: an observational study. *Quality and Safety in Health Care* 12(4): 273–9.

Braithwaite J, Runciman WB, Merry AF (2009) Towards safer, better healthcare: harnessing the natural properties of complex sociotechnical systems. *Quality and Safety in Health Care* 18(1): 37–41.

Briggs IM, Myers PB (1980) *Gifts Differing: Understanding Personality Type*. Mountain View, CA, Davies-Black Publishing.

Bronstein LR (2003) A model for interdisciplinary collaboration. *Social Work* 48(3): 297–306.

Buck MM, Tilson ER, Andersen JC (1999) Implementation and evaluation of an interdisciplinary health professions core curriculum. *Journal of Allied Health* 28(3): 174–8.

Declercq E, Barger M, Cabral H.J. *et al.* (2007) Maternal outcomes associated with planned primary cesarean births compared with planned vaginal births. *Obstetrics and Gynecology* 109(3): 669–77.

Department of Health (2000) *The NHS Plan: A Plan for Investment, A Plan for Reform*. London, HMSO.

Department of Health (2004) *National Service Framework for Children, Young People and Maternity Services*. London, Stationery Office. www.dh.gov.uk/en/Healthcare/Children/NationalServiceFrameworkdocuments/index.htm (accessed June, 2010).

Department of Health (2006a) *Our Health, Our Care, Our Say: A New Direction for Community Services.* London: Stationery Office. www.dh.gov.uk/en/Publicationsandstatistics/Publications/PublicationsPolicyAndGuidance/DH_4139925 (accessed June, 2010).

Department of Health (2006b) *In the Patient's Interest: Multi-professional Working Across Organisational Boundaries.* www.dh.gov.uk/en/Publicationsandstatistics/Publications/PublicationsPolicyAndGuidance/DH_4008963 (accessed June, 2010).

Department of Health (2007) *Maternity Matters: Choice, Access and Continuity of Care in a Safe Service.* www.dh.gov.uk/en/Publicationsandstatistics/Publications/PublicationsPolicyAndGuidance/DH_073312 (accessed June, 2010).

Donnison J (1977) *Midwives and Medical Men: A History of Inter-Professional Rivalries And Women's Rights.* New York, Schocken Books.

Dougherty MB, Larson E (2005) A review of instruments measuring nurse–physician collaboration. *Journal of Nursing Administration* 35(5): 244–53.

Downe S (2010) Beyond evidence-based medicine: complexity, and stories of maternity care. *Journal of Evaluation in Clinical Practice* 16(1): 232–7.

Downe S, McCourt C (2008) From being to becoming: reconstructing childbirth knowledges. In Downe S (ed) *Normal Birth, Evidence and Debate,* 2nd edn. Oxford, Elsevier.

Gieryn TF (1983) Boundary-work and the demarcation of science from non-science: strains and interests in professional ideologies of scientists. *American Sociological Review* 48: 781–95.

Goleman D (1995) *Emotional Intelligence: Why It Can Matter More Than IQ.* London, Bloomsbury.

Harris KT, Treanor CM, Salisbury ML (2006) Improving patient safety with team coordination: challenges and strategies of implementation. *Journal of Obstetrics, Gynecologic and Neonatal Nursing* 35(4): 557–66.

Health Care Commission (2006) Investigation into 10 maternal deaths at, or following delivery at, Northwick Park Hospital, North West London Hospitals NHS Trust, between April 2002 and April 2005. www.chi.gov.uk/_db/_documents/Northwick_tagged.pdf (accessed June, 2010).

Herzberg F (1964) The motivation–hygiene concept and problems of manpower. *Personnel Administration* January-February: 3–7.

Hodnett ED, Downe S, Edwards N, Walsh D (2005) Home-like versus conventional institutional settings for birth. *Cochrane Database of Systematic Reviews* 1: CD000012.

Hojat M, Fields SK, Veloski JJ, Griffiths M, Cohen MJ, Plumb JD (1999) Psychometric properties of an attitude scale measuring physician–nurse collaboration. *Evaluation and the Health Professions* 22(2): 208–20.

Hope JM, Lugassy D, Meyer R et al. (2005) Bringing interdisciplinary and multicultural team building to health care education: the Downstate Team-Building Initiative. *Academic Medicine* 80(1): 74–83.

Horak BJ, Pauig J, Keidan B, Kerns J (2004) Patient safety: a case study in team building and interdisciplinary collaboration. *Journal for Healthcare Quality* 26 (2): 6–12.

Hunter B (2004) Conflicting ideologies as a source of emotion work in midwifery. *Midwifery* 20(3): 261–72.

Kelly S, Allison MA (1998) *The Complexity Advantage*. New York, McGraw-Hill.

Kilsztajn S, Carmo MS, Machado LC Jr, Lopes ES, Lima LZ (2007) Caesarean sections and maternal mortality in Sao Paulo. *European Journal of Obstetrics and Gynecology and Reproductive Biology* 132(1): 64–9.

King's Fund (2008) *Safer Births: Everybody's Business.* www.kingsfund.org .uk/research/projects/improving_safety_in_maternity_services/ (accessed June, 2010).

Klein JT (2008) Evaluation of interdisciplinary and transdisciplinary research: a literature review. *American Journal of Preventive Medicine* 35(2 suppl): S116–23.

Leggat SG (2007) Teaching and learning teamwork: competency requirements for healthcare managers. *Journal of Health Administration Education* 24(2): 135–49.

Lemieux-Charles L, McGuire WL (2006) What do we know about health care team effectiveness? A review of the literature. *Medical Care Research and Review* 63(3): 263–300.

Lewin K (1951) *Field Theory in Social Science*. New York, Harper and Row.

Lewis G (ed) (2004) *Why Mothers Die 2000–2002*. The Sixth Report of the Confidential Enquiries into Maternal Deaths in the United Kingdom. London, Royal College of Obstetricians and Gynaecologists.

Lewis G (2007) *Saving Mothers' Lives: Reviewing Maternal Deaths to Make Motherhood Safer – 2003–2005*. The Seventh Report of the Confidential Enquiries into Maternal Deaths in the United Kingdom. London, CEMACH. www.cemach.org.uk/Publications/CEMACH-Publications/Maternal-and-Perinatal- Health.aspx (accessed June, 2010).

Lyndon A (2006) Communication and teamwork in patient care: how much can we learn from aviation? *Journal of Obstetric, Gynecologic and Neonatal Nursing* 35 (4): 538–46.

MacDorman MF, Declercq E, Menacker F, Malloy MH (2008) Neonatal mortality for primary cesarean and vaginal births to low-risk women: application of an "intention-to-treat" model. *Birth* 35(1): 3–8.

Machin D, Scamell M (1997) The experience of labour: using ethnography to explore the irresistible nature of the bio-medical metaphor during labour. *Midwifery* 13(2): 78–84.

Martin E (1987) *The Woman in the Body: A Cultural Analysis of Reproduction*. Boston, MA, Beacon Press.

Medical Research Council (2008) *Developing and Evaluating Complex Interventions: New Guidance*. www.mrc.ac.uk/Utilities/Documentrecord/ index.htm?d=MRC004871 (accessed June, 2010).

Miller S (1997) Midwives' and physicians' experiences in collaborative practice: a qualitative study. *Women's Health Issues* 7(5): 301–8.

National Childbirth Trust (2004) *Birth Services in Mid Sussex: What is Most Important to Women?* London, National Childbirth Trust.

National Health Service (2006) *NHS Leadership Qualities Framework: Collaborative Working,* p.31. www.NHSLeadershipQualities.nhs.uk (accessed June, 2010).

National Institute for Health and Clinical Excellence (2007) Clinical Guideline on Intrapartum Care: Management and Delivery of Care to Women in Labour. www.nice.org.uk/CG55 (accessed June, 2010).

Nicolescu B (2007) Transdisciplinarity – past, present and future. In Haverkort B, Reijntjes C (eds) *Moving Worldviews: Reshaping Sciences, Policies and Practices for Endogenous Sustainable Development.* Leusden, Netherlands, ETC/Compas, 142–66.

Nicolescu B (2009) *Disciplinary Boundaries.* Centre International de Recherches et Études Transdisciplinaires. http://basarab.nicolescu.perso.sfr.fr/ciret/ARTICLES/liste_articles.html (accessed June, 2010)

Oakley A (1985) *The Captured Womb: A History of the Medical Care of Pregnant Women.* London, Blackwell Publishers.

Pinki P, Sayasneh A, Lindow SW (2007) The working relationship between midwives and junior doctors: a questionnaire survey of Yorkshire trainees. *Journal of Obstetrics and Gynaecology* (4): 365–7.

Quinlivan JA, Black KI, Petersen RW, Kornman LH (2003) Differences in learning objectives during the labour ward clinical attachment between medical students and their midwifery preceptors. *Medical Education* 37: 913–20.

Redshaw M, Rowe R, Hockley C, Brocklehurst P (2007) *Recorded Delivery: A National Survey Of Women's Experience Of Maternity Care, 2006.* Oxford, National Perinatal Epidemiology Unit, University of Oxford.

Reeves S, Zwarenstein M, Goldman J. *et al.* (2008) Interprofessional education: effects on professional practice and health care outcomes. *Cochrane Database of Systematic Reviews* 1: CD002213.

Reeves S, Rice K, Conn LG, Miller KL, Kenaszchuk C, Zwarenstein M (2009) Interprofessional interaction, negotiation and non-negotiation on general internal medicine wards. *Journal of Interprofessional Care* 20: 1–13.

Reiger KM, Lane KL (2009) Working together: collaboration between midwives and doctors in public hospitals. *Australian Health Review* 33(2): 315–24.

Salovey P, Mayer JD (1990) Emotional intelligence. *Imagination, Cognition, and Personality* 9: 185–211.

Simpson KR, James DC, Knox GE (2006) Nurse–physician communication during labor and birth: implications for patient safety. *Journal of Obstetric, Gynecologic and Neonatal Nursing* 35(4): 547–56.

Star SL, Griesemer JR (1989) Institutional ecology, 'translations' and boundary objects: amateurs and professionals in Berkeley's Museum of Vertebrate Zoology, 1907–39. *Social Studies of Science* 19(4): 387–420.

Swanson EA, Taylor CM, Valentine AM, McCarthy AM (1998) The integrated health professions education program seminar. *Nurse Education* 23(2): 18–21.

Tuckman BW (2001) Developmental sequence in small groups. *Group Facilitation* Spring. http://findarticles.com/p/articles/mi_qa3954/is_200104/ai_n8943663/?tag=content;col1 (accessed June, 2010).

Weisman CS, Gordon DL, Cassard SD, Bergner M, Wong R (1993) The effects of unit self-management on hospital nurses' work process, work satisfaction, and retention. *Medical Care* 31(5): 381–93.

Weiss SJ, Davis HP (1985) Validity and reliability of the Collaborative Practice Scales. *Nursing Research* 34(5): 299–305.

Wenger E (ed) (1998) *Communities of Practice: Learning, Meaning, and Identity.* Cambridge, Cambridge University Press.

Wenger E, McDermott RA, Snyder W (2002) *Cultivating Communities of Practice: A Guide to Managing Knowledge.* Boston, MA, Harvard Business School Press.

Wood DJ, Gray B (1991) Toward a comprehensive theory of collaboration. *Journal of Applied Behavioral Science* 27: 139–62.

Zwarenstein M, Bryant W (2000) Interventions to promote collaboration between nurses and doctors. *Cochrane Database of Systematic Reviews* 2: CD000072.

Zwarenstein M, Goldman J, Reeves S (2009) Interprofessional collaboration: effects of practice-based interventions on professional practice and healthcare outcomes. *Cochrane Database of Systematic Reviews* 4: CD000072.

Chapter 10
Case Studies of Collaboration in the UK and China

Ngai Fen Cheung and Anita Fleming

Introduction

This chapter explores collaborative activities in the UK and China, as illustrations of the theories set out in Chapter 9. Collaborations, either in research or in practice, are built on mutual understanding of each other's role and responsibility (AAM 2004) and these case studies describe how such understandings can be developed and sustained.

Previous studies have discussed principles for collaborative activities in order to improve health outcomes, the quality of the services and cost-effectiveness. The nature of these principles can be summed up as 'to be open to' and 'to share in' the activities which are deemed to be essential in collaborative working in midwifery, and also in other professions and disciplines where collaboration is taking place. The activities that should be 'open' include communication, discussion, mutual trust, respect, understanding and support. Those that should be 'shared' are information, value, vision, power, responsibility, accountability and team decision making (Keleher 1998; McPherson *et al.* 2001; AAM 2004; DH 2007). While the list may constitute ideal types of good or effective collaboration, they are by no means unproblematic, nor are they the only aspects essential to collaboration. There is also the question of equality. This refers to the different standing of partners, including social and cultural attributes. It also refers to relations with those using the services. In China, for instance, while multidisciplinary teams are almost a routine in maternity care, cross-cultural collaborations are also

Essential Midwifery Practice: Leadership, Expertise and Collaborative Working, first edition. Edited by Soo Downe, Sheena Byrom and Louise Simpson
Published 2011 by Blackwell Publishing Ltd.
© 2011 Blackwell Publishing Ltd.

becoming increasingly important if midwives are to enhance their vision by understanding maternity care under diverse social and cultural conditions.

Collaboration can be either hierarchical or non-hierarchical. This begs the question of whether all things that should be shared are in fact shared in specific collaborations. For example, who holds the resources? In a cross-cultural situation, shared values can also be problematic. It is most likely that resources and values are distributed unequally. This means that effective collaboration might be measured by the degree to which 'openness' and 'share' are operational, rather than looking for absolute equality. The relative success of this depends on the motivations, social expectations and commitments of each participant (Rex 1961).

A collaborative research project to set up a midwife-led normal birth unit (MNBU) with educational and maternity care institutions in China revealed some problems of 'openness' and 'share'. These will be discussed later in this chapter, along with other issues relating to multidisciplinary and departmental collaboration in the Chinese setting.

First, however, we present two specific case studies of collaboration in maternity care. These have emerged from the work undertaken by midwives and obstetricians in East Lancashire Hospitals Trust. The trust is based in the north west of England and includes two hospital sites, and also provides a community midwifery and a home birth service. A midwifery caseholding group provides continuity of carer to women with specific clinical and psychosocial needs. There are over 6000 births a year across the trust, and the population sociodemographics range from some of the most deprived to some of the wealthiest groups in the UK. There is a varied ethnic mix, with the main groups being those of White British and those of South Asian origin. The population geography ranges from densely urban to remote rural communities. The case studies demonstrate how good collaborative partnerships, in these cases between midwives and obstetricians, improve birth experiences for women.

Collaboration in East Lancashire, England

The first case study describes a situation in which a midwife referred to an obstetrician. The second case, in contrast, involves an obstetrician referring to a midwife for input and support. Both situations were based on the aim of maximising the woman's chance of experiencing a positive birth. This demonstrates how effective collaboration involves a two-way respect and understanding, and it demonstrates both the openness and the sharing criteria described above.

Case study 1 – midwife referring to obstetrician

Mrs A was pregnant with her second baby, and after having experienced a traumatic birth experience with her first baby, resulting in an emergency caesarean section, requested a home birth supported by midwives. At the outset, she declined any input from doctors whatsoever. The reason behind this was that she felt that the outcomes of the previous labour were due to the fact that there had been too much medical intervention, and she hadn't been listened to. She had felt helpless and disempowered.

Mrs A was an educated and well-read woman, who listened to, and also researched herself, the risks of vaginal birth after caesarean section. She agreed to speak to a supervisor of midwives regarding these issues, to ensure she had up-to-date and evidence-based information to make fully informed choices. Her views and wishes remained unchanged, however, with regard to being under the care of an obstetrician. She was subsequently supported throughout her pregnancy by the local caseholding group of midwives, who she came to know very well.

In the first pregnancy, Mrs A had felt pressured to have her labour induced because of postmaturity, and because a large baby was anticipated. She felt that this was the beginning of the whole cascade of intervention. She was adamant that she would not be induced for those reasons in this pregnancy. As her pregnancy approached term, it was evident that this was going to be another large baby, and the midwife raised the issue of exploring the options should there be any complications again. As Mrs A had developed a trusting relationship with the midwives by this stage, and felt that they would support her wishes and not make excuses for her to go to hospital without a valid reason, she listened to the suggestion of the midwife.

The midwife reassured Mrs A that her home birth would continue to be supported, but suggested that it would be useful to have the opportunity to discuss options with an understanding and supportive obstetrician, to agree a plan as back-up should everything not progress smoothly. Mrs A was quite anxious about this, as she felt that the obstetrician would try to frighten her into going to hospital and would pressure her into undergoing intervention that she did not really want to have. Despite these concerns, she agreed to attend the appointment, supported by her midwife.

At the appointment the obstetrician, as expected, explained the evidence around the risks and benefits of vaginal birth after caesarean section, particularly with regard to giving birth at home, but then documented that she felt that Mrs A had a good understanding of the issues and that she was making fully informed choices. The obstetrician then went on to say that, hopefully, everything would go well with the labour and birth, but that it would be good to explore the options should that not be the case in order to keep mother and baby as safe as possible. She offered access to her should complications occur at any time, and also offered additional monitoring in the form of ultrasound scans for liquor volume and CTG monitoring should the pregnancy go beyond term +14 days. In addition to this, a plan was agreed and documented in the hospital records with regard to management of a caesarean section should it be required, this being due to the fact that certain aspects of the care during Mrs A's first caesarean section had resulted in her being particularly upset.

Mrs A left the appointment feeling surprisingly well supported by an obstetrician and while she remained confident that she would have a straightforward normal birth at home, she also felt reassured that should problems occur, she need not be frightened of having to go into hospital.

In the event, Mrs A's pregnancy continued to term +19 days. She accepted the offer of the obstetrician to be monitored after term +14 days. She started in labour spontaneously and remained at home for most of the labour. However, labour progress slowed towards the later first stage and, eventually, she agreed to be transferred into hospital. Eventually, she agreed with the midwife and the obstetrician that she and her baby probably needed a caesarean section. This was undertaken very sensitively and, in the end, she felt very happy and positive about the birth experience and outcome. She felt that she had been fully supported in her choices and, more importantly, had been involved in all decisions that were made. Along with her midwife, she had agreed that it was the right time to transfer to hospital, and with the obstetrician they had all agreed that it was the right time to have a caesarean section. This had been conducted in the way it had been agreed and documented in her records. So, despite having a second caesarean section, Mrs A actually felt that her birth was a positive and empowering experience, and that this was due to good partnership working of the whole team, including herself. This illustrates clear efforts across the collaborating parties (including the woman) to be open, to share, and to equalise resources of knowledge and power, for the well-being and safety of the mother and her baby.

Case study 2 – obstetrician referring to midwife

Mrs B was also pregnant with her second baby. She had also experienced a previous traumatic birth for her first baby, following induction of labour with a consequent caesarean section.

However, in contrast to Mrs A, she had sought the care of an obstetrician from the outset, and requested that she have an elective caesarean section this time, as she felt she could not go through the trauma again that she had experienced the first time.

The obstetrician had assured Mrs B that she would support her choices, but suggested referral to a caseload midwife who would be the named midwife during the pregnancy, birth and postnatal period. During the referral communication with the midwife, the obstetrician suggested that, with good midwifery and support, Mrs B might develop the confidence to try to achieve a normal birth.

As with Mrs A, a relationship built on trust and respect developed through the pregnancy. This enabled the events of her previous birth to be explored and discussed. Mrs B had chosen to have an epidural in the first labour, and after that, progress had slowed down. A syntocinon infusion had been commenced, and was consequently increased, and then fetal distress developed which led to the decision to perform a caesarean section. Discussions between the midwife and Mrs B included the advantages and disadvantages of epidural analgesia in labour, including the effect on mobilisation and ability to adapt different positions, and also around how to work with pain in labour to try to minimise the need for epidural analgesia and pharmacological drugs. By 36 weeks of pregnancy Mrs B became much more confident and began to waver in her decision to have an elective caesarean section. She felt that she really wanted to try for a normal birth, but still had reservations. What if she tried for a normal birth but developed complications in labour and changed her mind? And what if she decided to try for a normal birth but then didn't start labour spontaneously, as she did not want to be induced again?

An appointment was made for Mrs B, her husband and her midwife to see the obstetrician together to discuss the options. Following this, a plan was agreed. Mrs B would plan to have a normal birth, but it was documented in the records that if complications arose during the labour, she could go straight for caesarean section instead of other interventions being attempted first. The other agreement made was that if the pregnancy progressed to term + 14 days, then a caesarean section could be offered instead of induction of labour if this is what Mrs B still wished at that time.

All involved were happy with the decisions and the agreed plan. As the pregnancy had gone well, and the baby was in a good position, the obstetrician and midwife were confident that Mrs B had a good chance of the labour progressing. Mrs B felt confident to try for a normal birth, with the reassurance that there was an agreed plan in place should there be any problems.

In the event, Mrs B went into spontaneous labour at term + 3 days. She rang the midwife when her contractions became regular and agreed to meet her at the hospital. On the way to hospital the contractions quickly became very strong and close together. Mrs B was fully dilated on admission to hospital, and had a normal birth very soon afterwards. She was really pleased that she had chosen not just to opt directly for the elective section, and was thrilled at the outcome.

These two case studies demonstrate how positive collaborative relationships, based on mutual respect and understanding of each other's roles, can make a huge difference to a woman's birth experience.

Collaboration in China

In this section, Ngai Fen Cheung describes the development of collaborative partnerships which ultimately led to the successful establishment of China's first midwife-led birth unit (MNBU).

Demise of Chinese midwifery

In 1993, the Chinese government decided that midwifery was no longer a profession in birthing care and formal midwifery education was discontinued in the urban areas. In the decade that followed, former midwives were phasing out and losing their professional identity. This was followed by state legislation in 2003 which proposed a target of 100% of births in China taking place in hospital. The proposal suggested that birth would be 'safer' though not necessarily natural. As in similar legislative moves elsewhere in the world, this could be seen as an overambitious and erroneous project driven by modern 'technocratic values' (Davis-Floyd *et al.* 2009).

By this point, medical authorities were firmly established in attending births in China. A rapid development of a market economy in all areas of life had led to a hard-wired economic and technological rationality for many civil and societal processes. Efficiency in quantitative and monetary terms was what was to be achieved, even in such natural life processes as giving birth. It became practically a fashion for healthy women with a normal pregnancy in Chinese urban areas to opt for caesarean sections. All of this happened against the background of the prevalent birth control policies then in China. As births became less important to society, so midwifery practice became more of a thing of the past.

Collaborative research into Chinese midwifery

The Chinese experience was not unprecedented. Midwifery in most industrialised countries has been kept under the shadow of medical authority up until very recently. The general world experiences of midwifery only differ in degree from that of Chinese midwifery, in that, in most countries, a formal professional identity of midwifery, and midwifery education provision, has not vanished altogether. The disciplinary relation between midwifery and the social sciences in the UK may have given midwives some insight into understanding the importance of the leading roles of midwives in maternity care to promote natural births. The idea of the MNBU came into being in the UK in the 1990s, but it was still very much an ideal and unusual setting for maternity care as midwifery entered the new millennium (Walsh 2007).

It may seem to be self-evident that if China moves down along the industrial path taken before by western European countries, it will develop childbirth systems that mirror those of the latter. But China is culturally and socially different from Europe. While some values from the West may help the Chinese to transform economically, the childbirth models that work there will not necessarily translate effectively into Chinese practices.

One way of exploring this issue is to set up collaborative cross-cultural research. In pursuit of this ideal, a small collaboration was started in 2004 between an important maternity hospital in Shanghai, China, and the School of Health in the Social Sciences at the University of Edinburgh, UK. The work was funded by the British Academy, the University of Edinburgh and the Chinese institution. Maternity hospitals and units in eastern and southern China were visited by the research team from Edinburgh, and interviews were carried out by both the Chinese and the British research teams. The collaboration enabled us to explore each other's birthing practices (Cheung *et al.* 2005a, b; 2006a, b; Mander & Cheung 2006). A collaborative research partnership was established in 2007 between the College of Nursing of the Hangzhou Normal University in eastern China and the School of Health of the University of Edinburgh, to set up an MNBU in a Chinese hospital. The project has been supported by the Carnegie Trust, the Royal Society of Edinburgh and the Chinese city council of Hangzhou. Midwifery academics, midwives, the nursing education authority, doctors and the hospital care authorities came together to negotiate for the setting up of such a unit. The negotiation established the inspiration of the MNBU in promoting normal birth and in reviving Chinese midwifery. This collaborative process revealed that academic leadership is an important element in collaboration. This is because of the intellectual and persuasive capacity that academic institutions can demonstrate.

As midwifery had been phased out in China since the 1990s, it appeared that even a collaborative research study into midwifery practices would certainly be out of the question, not to mention setting up a midwife-led unit. But the remaining hope was that China remains a literary country in which innovation and intellectual development are still very much respected.

Starting collaboration in midwifery research and practice in China also came after the notorious SARS epidemic in 2003, when healthcare problems were very much on the Chinese national agenda (WHO 2004). Our midwifery collaborative research proposals were getting quick responses in 2004 and 2007, firstly through personal academic relationships and later through university employment. The MNBU project in

China was a collaborative study between three institutions from two different countries: the UK and China. There were great social, cultural and linguistic barriers to overcome. To enhance cross-cultural vision in maternity care, midwifery researchers are required to be trained in understanding different cultures.

One of the problems we encountered in the institutional collaboration was a 'level of scholarship' between institutions. The question was raised first by the University of Edinburgh (UE). The university has many of its academic disciplines rated as internationally excellent, including midwifery and the social sciences. The institutional leads were concerned about the scholarly capacity that the collaborating university in China had. The Chinese college of nursing, which had just amalgamated into a new city university, needed to form its own scholarly base. Collaboration with the University of Edinburgh was certainly a good opportunity to do so. To collaborate or not to collaborate became the question for the UE, not so much as a moral obligation to help as a practical decision to extend knowledge, and the sphere of scholarly interest. While the importance of equal scholarly capacity is clear in some areas of academic achievement, it was less obvious to the collaborating partners that this was important in the current circumstances, when the collaboration was set up to learn with and from each other, and to create a bridge (in this case via cross-cultural personnel) for the learning to take place. Of course, there can be a difference in intellectual resources, which could be an element in efficient collaboration, but which can also either be shared or manipulated.

The first hospital in China we approached was a teaching hospital attached to the faculty of medicine in our collaborative university. When we approached it regarding the possibility of the MNBU project, the hospital was concerned about the 'intellectual property' of the project before the work was even started. The value of 'intellectual property' has now been legitimised thanks to the rationale of the global market economy. Although the tide seemed to have turned in Chinese healthcare so that there was a more favourable attitude towards the MNBU project, medical-led maternity care is still entrenched in China. Such a firm belief was behind the concern about 'intellectual property' by our collaborator to be, who chaired the maternity unit in the hospital and who was a locally renowned obstetric consultant. As there was a supposed 'intellectual hierarchy' existing between doctors and midwives, this necessarily lead to the question of who should take the lead in claiming the 'intellectual property' that might result from collaboration. It was a naive but manipulative proposition, which might amount to a kind of 'collaboration hijacking'. We duly withdrew from the negotiation, and set the project up with a different hospital.

Collaboration between women, their families and the midwife

China's first MNBU became operational in March 2008. It is known locally as '温馨产房 (homely birthplace)'. The unit consists of a mixed skill team of four junior and eight senior midwives rotating on shifts, and three midwifery managers. Apart from supervising the juniors in the MNBU, the senior midwives are also responsible for the supervision of the standard care unit and liaison with obstetricians if any abnormality occurs. The job of the three midwifery managers is to supervise and co-ordinate all the activities and care in the maternity unit which includes the labour unit, the antenatal and postnatal wards in the hospital.

Seven hundred and seventy eight people took part in the MNBU study. They were 178 midwives, 507 women, 88 birth companions and five obstetricians. The study featured midwife-led care, a birth plan, complementary therapies and 'two-to-one' care from a midwife and birth companion of the woman's choice. Such care was not identified elsewhere in China. The vaginal birth rate was 87.6% in the MNBU compared with 58.8% in standard care. All participating women were happy to have given birth there. The concept of having both a support person and a midwife with the labouring women (two-to-one care, as above) emerged as a fundamental factor of the woman's experience, and of effective utilisation of midwives' skills. Medical practitioners felt that the unit facilitated women's understanding and compliance if transferred. Pain control and episiotomy utilisation need further study, as do perceptions of staff shortages.

The higher rate of vaginal birth and lower rate of caesarean in the MNBU are significant. These cannot be achieved without the model of two-to-one care, which encourages women and midwives' active collaboration in the care of childbirth. The social relationship of the midwife and of the birth companion is regarded as a means of achieving a desirable birthing experience for the mother. The physical being with the woman and ritualistic or symbolic presence raises a point for the analysis of social and midwifery supporting system, which indicates a holistic philosophy rather than health professional orientation.

Collaboration between midwives

Because of their lower social status when compared to doctors, Chinese midwives have been fighting a losing battle, especially in collaborative work. The hospital midwives were keen to participate in this project, as they saw that it would enhance their role and clinical practice. They recognised the project's potential for them to regain their former functions and status. Thus, the midwives in this unit grasped the opportunity presented to them. They realised that for too long the Chinese midwife had been marginalised with directly negative consequences for midwives and childbearing women. These consequences are particularly evident in the phenomenally high caesarean rates in many areas in China (Cheung *et al.* 2005b).

Working within the MNBU provides an environment where the midwives can practise to the full extent of the role. This is cost-effective and allows time for them to provide care to women in labour. The role of the labour ward co-ordinator is to ensure that support can be provided to staff across the whole department. The unit managed to achieve higher rates of satisfaction and vaginal births compared with those of the standard care unit. This empowers Chinese midwives to regain their lost profession.

Multiprofessional collaboration

The collaborations built up through an early research project into caesarean section decision making in China, and during the development and evaluation of the MNBU, illustrate the process of knowledge and relationship transformation in maternity care in specific Chinese settings (Cheung *et al.* 2005a, b; 2006a, b; Mander & Cheung 2006; Cheung *et al.* 2009a, b; Mander *et al.* 2010). The professionals involved were researchers, midwives, obstetricians, nurses, heads of departments, and the head of the hospitals. These two completed projects taught us that the collaborative working experience of multiprofessionals was achieved through teamwork, researchers' personality and their appropriate relationship with the right people, in the right places and at the right time.

We had to decide how to relate to each other in new and changing circumstances. Sometimes these changes had come about unplanned as a result of forces under no one's control, for example, shortage of midwives. Other situations in which people have tried to find their way have been the consequence of deliberate policies of reformers and revolutionaries, determined to reconstruct the ways in which people act in relation to each other. For example, before the studies, midwives were not allowed to discharge women from hospital. This issue had to be addressed before the work could continue.

Reality is not created by purely rational forms of action. Augmentation of labour was frequently used in the MNBU and the obstetric unit (OU) in our study. This was perceived as necessary because of a conviction among the health workers that interventions such as oxytocic administration and amniotomy could shorten the duration of labour and resolve the problem of a serious shortage of staff. In the MNBU the initial persistence of this conviction led to the midwives using these interventions if a woman's labour was expected to continue into the night, when staffing was perceived as particularly inadequate.

Episiotomy was also frequently used in both groups of the randomised controlled trial of 226 women in our study. Having said this, there was a significant difference between the units with 77.9% (n = 176) of women in the MNBU having an episiotomy as opposed to nearly 94.2% (n = 131 versus 139 cases of vaginal births apart from those giving birth by caesarean) in the OU. The frequency of episiotomy implies that it is a routine prophylactic intervention, especially in the standard care setting. Despite having informed the midwives of the research evidence, the midwives experienced genuine difficulty in letting go of this routine intervention.

Rationally, the health workers have to work within the norms as perceived by the maternity team. The capacity to change this collaboratively may reflect a threefold lack of confidence. Firstly, the midwives lacked confidence in their own ability to limit perineal damage and relied too much on their medical colleagues. Secondly, the midwives doubted the women's abilities to co-operate sufficiently to limit trauma to the perineum. And thirdly, there was a fear of a third-degree perineal tear or genital tears which may have been compounded by litigation anxiety, resulting in what the midwives considered to be a defensive form of practice. Irrationally, despite all the evidence, obstetric interventions are still widely used among healthy women, based on a range of non-evidence based reasons.

Overcoming operational conflict

As a result of development and evolution, there is an increasing recognition of the midwife's role, retrospectively or prospectively, in the Chinese system. Such an interest in the midwife's role is in conflict with the existing obstetric-led maternity care. The time has come for a reconstruction of the structure through separation, partition, redistribution or reanalysing the structure. Such an interest in the structure has now developed into the MNBU in which a midwife is designated to take care of a woman. This arrangement has led not only to greater consistency and better planned care but also the formation of deeper working relationships, which have led to better care. In theory, the development of the MNBU and changes made in the management could lead to conflict between obstetricians and midwives as obstetric care is still the mainstream in China. This is one of the conflicts that we call an 'operational conflict', which can occur within a structure at some stage of its development or evolution. 'Operational conflict' can affect effective collaboration between midwives and obstetricians.

In fact, the presence of the MNBU and its services in Hangzhou has been very well received by the service users and service providers. The emergence of the MNBU is a reorganisation of the maternity care structure that explicitly recognises the midwife's role in the system. While this could have led to conflict, in this case, it increased doctor–midwife collaboration in care, as we shall discuss below. It created an alteration of the existing maternity care structure into one in which midwifery care and obstetric care have an overlapping rather than an overseeing relationship. This has meant that the MNBU has reshaped the structure of the services and redistributed the power of clinical decision making to midwives and opened up other possibilities. The development of the MNBU has eased the 'operational conflict', but one may argue that it will also bring about 'interest conflict' functionally in the new system as it means obstetricians have lost their total control or even jobs they used to enjoy in the old system. Such an 'interest conflict' would again hinder effective collaboration between midwives and obstetricians.

Is there an 'interest conflict'? In the British maternity care system, as demonstrated in the East Lancashire case studies above, there are now agreed guidelines between obstetricians and midwives (NHS Institute 2006). While this may be a 'political correction', it nevertheless indicates that a common interest can exist between doctors and midwives. The Chinese case has shown a more complicated picture. The establishment of the MNBU has affected both the workloads and financial incentives in the Chinese hospital. All the obstetricians interviewed said that they felt relieved of the workload pressure after the MNBU was established. In this case, an 'interest conflict' did not arise. On the other hand, women pay less in the MNBU than they do under obstetric care, while receiving services which they thought were of high quality. This means a loss of income for the hospital as a financial unit under the healthcare system in China. In this case, the other departments would look upon the MNBU as a loser in terms of the profit the hospital could make. The fact that we have not heard such a complaint so far does not necessarily mean that there is not such a complaint or 'interest conflict'. Quite often in Chinese hospitals, it is the quest for increasing profits that encourages questionable medical interventions, including ordering needless tests, intravenous infusions, performing unnecessary caesarean sections and forceps deliveries, and overly prescribing medications. The health workers have a direct interest in the tests and procedures they order.

In the case of the MNBU study, it was fortunate that the heads of the hospital and the departments were able to recognise that the care should be motivated by a concern for people rather than profits. In addition, the MNBU project was funded by the city government. As the project had been authorised, the shortfall in the income of the staff working in the MNBU was met by the funding and the hospital financial authority, who were able to harmonise the financial relationship between departments. As this issue was overcome, it has not been a factor in creating an 'interest conflict' between the doctors and the midwives. Indeed, the effect of the MNBU may just be like a stone dropping in a pond whose ripples would lap the existing collaborative web.

The separation between obstetrician care and midwifery care in the maternity care system should be a functional one, not a structural one. They can be seen as co-existing in a maternity care structure. This argument is reflected in a recent British NHS document in which it is stipulated that 'midwife-led care does not depend on physical boundaries' (NHS Institute 2006). In other words, the separation between obstetrician care and midwifery care is not a physical one, since they all work within the same structure of maternity care. But a physical separation between the doctors and the midwives in the Chinese MNBU case, in which obstetricians are not allowed to enter the unit unless invited, has proved to be a technique to achieve the structural alteration. The technique should be seen as contextualised in the Chinese setting where midwifery was on the brink of extinction. Ironically, modern obstetric technology is still largely unavailable to the majority of Chinese, especially in the rural areas, but the more it is not available, the more it is in great demand. The physical separation of the first MNBU in the maternity care setting in China is intended to have the effect of maximising well-being for women and babies, limiting the demand for unnecessary obstetric intervention, and reinstating midwifery practice.

Conclusion

The projects and case studies described and discussed in this chapter demonstrate that positive collaborative partnerships are in operation and being further developed in both China and the UK. Although these may be at different stages of progress and set in different historical, cultural and political contexts, it is evident that the creation of mutual respect and trust, the input of strong and effective leadership, and the ability to positively influence others through the development of innovative practices are essential to this process. Many of the characteristics and attributes described in Chapter 9 are in evidence in these case studies. They are all a work in progress. However, continuation of a desire to be open to others, and to share economic and moral resources suggests that they may move the local service in each case towards increased collaboration, and better outcomes for women, babies, families, and the staff themselves. If they can be replicated in other settings, the underlying principles of these projects may also form a basis for effective change in maternity care within and between regions, and even countries.

References

Alberta Association of Midwives (AAM) (2004) *Guidelines for the Collaborative Working Relationship Between Registered Midwives and Registered Nurses.* www. nurses.ab.ca/Carna-Admin/Uploads/Midwives%20and%20RNs.pdf (accessed June, 2010).

Cheung NF, Mander R, Cheng L, Yang XQ, Chen VY (2005a) Informed choice in the context of caesarean decision-making in China. *Evidence Based Midwifery* 3: 33–8.

Cheung NF, Mander R, Cheng L (2005b) The 'doula-midwives' in Shanghai. *Evidence Based Midwifery* 3: 73–9.

Cheung NF, Mander R, Cheng L. *et al.* (2006a) 'Zuoyuezi' after caesarean in China: an interview survey. *International Journal of Nursing Studies* 43: 193–202.

Cheung NF, Mander R, Cheng L, Yang XQ, Chen VY (2006b) Caesarean decision-making: negotiation between Chinese women and healthcare professionals. *Evidence Based Midwifery* 4: 24–30.

Cheung NF, Mander R, Wang X, Fu W, Zhu J (2009a) Chinese midwives' views on a midwife-led normal birth unit (MNBU). *Midwifery* 25(6): 744–55.

Cheung NF, Mander R, Wang X, Fu W, Zhu J (2009b) The planning and preparation for a 'homely birthplace' in Hangzhou, China. *Evidence Based Midwifery* 7(3): 101–6.

Davis-Floyd RB, Barclay B, Tritten J (2009) *Birth Models That Work.* Berkeley, CA, University of California Press.

Department of Health (2007) *Maternity Matters: Choice, Access and Continuity of Care in a Safe Service.* www.northwest.nhs.uk/document_uploads/ Maternity_Matters/DH_074199%5B1%5D.pdf (accessed June, 2010).

Keleher K (1998) Collaborative practice: characteristics, barriers, benefits, and implications for midwifery. *Journal of Nurse-Midwifery* 43(1): 8–11.

Mander R, Cheung NF (2006) Issues arising in the planning of a cross-cultural research project in China. *Clinical Effectiveness in Nursing* 9(suppl 2): e212–e220.

Mander R, Cheung NF, Wang X, Fu W, Zhu J (2010) Beginning an action research project to establish a midwife-led normal birthing unit in China. *Journal of Clinical Nursing* 19(3–4): 517–26.

McPherson K, Headrick L, Moss F (2001) Working and learning together: good quality care depends on it, but how can we achieve it? *Quality in Health Care* 10 (suppl2): ii46–ii53.

NHS, Institute for Innovation and Improvement (2006) *Delivering Quality and Value: Focus on Caesarean.* www.institute.nhs.uk/option,com_joomcart/ Itemid,26/main_page,document_product_info/products_id,185.html (accessed June, 2010).

Rex J (1961) *Key Problems of Sociological Theory.* London, Routledge and Kegan Paul.

Walsh D (2007) *Improving Maternity Services. Small is Beautiful – Lessons from a Birthing Centre.* Oxford, Radcliffe Publishing, 1–4.

World Health Organization (2004) *Country Cooperation Strategy: WHO China, Strategic Priorities for 2004–2008.* www.wpro.who.int/NR/rdonlyres/ E8FE334A-BAF5-49ED-89CC-BFE163F63C02/0/CCbook_eng.pdf (accessed June, 2010).

Chapter 11
Using Collaborative Theories to Reduce Caesarean Section Rates and Improve Maternal and Infant Well-being

Alison Brodrick, Nicky Mason, Janet Baldwin and Sophie Cowley

Introduction

This chapter describes how collaborative working contributed to the development of a toolkit to reduce unnecessary caesarean section rates. The project at the centre of the chapter was set up by the NHS Institute for Innovation and Improvement (NHS Institute). Its role is to 'support the NHS to transform healthcare for patients and the public by rapidly developing and spreading new ways of working, new technology and world class leadership' (NHS Institute 2009a). Work processes place a strong emphasis on collaborative working with other NHS organisations and staff to ensure that solutions which are developed meet the needs of those using them (NHS Institute 2009b). The caesarean section (CS) team at the NHS Institute has been working with maternity services in England since 2006 to promote normal birth, and reduce caesarean section rates. The work has comprised three phases, all of which involved the use of collaborative strategies.

- The development of the *Focus On: Caesarean Section* document (NHS Institute 2006a), working with nine maternity units in England.
- Piloting and development of the *Pathways to Success: A Self-Improvement Toolkit: Focus on Normal Birth and Reducing CS Rates* (NHS Institute 2007).

Essential Midwifery Practice: Leadership, Expertise and Collaborative Working, first edition. Edited by Soo Downe, Sheena Byrom and Louise Simpson Published 2011 by Blackwell Publishing Ltd.
© 2011 Blackwell Publishing Ltd.

- A national Spread and Adopt Programme, offering a programme of regional network events to all maternity services in England, and a focused support programme with 20 maternity units across England, to evaluate practice and facilitate change.

The *Pathways to Success* toolkit was developed through an ongoing collaborative process between the CS team, clinicians and stakeholders. In this chapter we discuss the collaborative approach taken by the CS team to develop the methodologies within the toolkit to support collaborative working. We also present the evidence that its use supports collaborative working within maternity services. We describe the implementation and impact of the Spread and Adopt Programme that followed the creation of the toolkit.

Whilst the original work of the NHS Institute was entitled *Focus On: Caesarean Section*, it quickly became apparent that, in order to reduce CS rates, clinicians must promote and encourage normality. This shift in practice is supported in the UK by government, professional organisations and consumer groups (National Childbirth Trust/Royal College of Midwives/Royal College of Obstetricians and Gynaecologists 2007). Achievement of this aim requires a collaborative and cohesive approach, both nationally and locally, between the professional organisations and women using the service. This focus on increased collaboration has been part of a range of recent health reforms as discussed below.

Reforming the NHS through increasing collaboration

In 2000 the English National Health Service (NHS) was set a challenging agenda for health reform in the *NHS Plan* (DH 2000). Following public consultation, this plan promised modernisation of the health service, with the aim of services being designed around the needs of the patient. Reform was to be accompanied by investment and a change in the relationship between the Department of Health and the NHS. As modernisation took place, greater control was given to local health economies, and there was a promise of more autonomy for front-line staff. The policy document recognised the need to set national standards and provide national support to deliver service changes and monitor the impact of reform at national level. This led to the establishment of the National Institute of Clinical Excellence (NICE), the NHS Modernisation Agency (MA) and the Commission for Health Improvement (CHI). Although largely funded by the Department of Health, these were independent organisations, whose role was to work with and through NHS organisations.

Much of this reform was characterised by a need for a change in relationships. Examples of increased collaboration include closer working with patients through the development of patient forums and patient advocates, increased sharing of clinical responsibility between professional disciplines through the extension of consultant nurse and midwife roles, and working across traditional organisational boundaries, including the integration of health and social care through (primary) care trusts (DH 2000).

Now, nearly 1-years after *The NHS Plan* and 60 years since the inception of the service in 1948, the NHS has undergone its largest review ever. This work was led for the government by Lord Ara Darzi, a health minister and a practising surgeon within the NHS, and included a remit to 'directly engage patients, NHS staff and the public' to ensure that 'a properly resourced NHS is clinically led, patient centred and locally accountable' (House of Commons 2007). This approach to a more inclusive and collaborative vision of what constitutes a 'world-class health service' is evidenced by an interim report, *Our NHS, Our Future* (DH 2007a). This document is based on conversations and meetings with thousands of patients, staff and the public. It captures their views on what they want of their NHS. Publication during the review process was intended to encourage ongoing public involvement, and to publicise the way in which people could participate in the subsequent stages of the review (DH 2007a). Each strategic health authority (SHA) has now also published its own vision and operating framework for making *High Quality Care for All* a reality (DH 2008).

At policy level, there is a strong steer for collaboration in healthcare design and development, with quality, innovation, productivity and prevention (QIPP) being both the latest drivers for and the key measures of improvement. Evolving from the NHS Modernisation Agency, the NHS Institute for Innovation and Improvement provides support to the NHS and NHS organisations. Greater involvement with healthcare reform at all levels is particularly evident in maternity service reform.

Maternity reforms and collaboration

In the UK, there is a long-standing history of collaboration between maternity care professionals and the women and families who use maternity services. This has shaped the current services and brought about considerable reform. The seminal *Changing Childbirth* report (DH 1993) highlighted the importance of developing positive relationships between women and clinicians by focusing on continuity of care through continuity of carer. The more recent *Maternity Matters* report (DH 2007b) brings choice to the forefront, with a set of national guarantees that provide opportunities for women and their families to explore options for care through discussion with their clinicians and carers. Safety has also featured highly in reports (Lewis 2007; O'Neill 2008) and is a crucial component in ensuring that maternity services are fit for purpose. Equally important is the quality of the woman's journey through the service. In this context, the issues of choice and collaboration feature highly. 'Patient' experience and engagement is one of five national priorities for 2009–10 for the NHS in England (DH/ NHS Finance 2008). Other indications of greater collaboration can be seen in the wide range of stakeholders who contribute to national clinical guidelines or are part of nominated guideline groups (NICE 2007). Many directives are now jointly produced by a range of professionals and user groups (National Childbirth Trust/Royal College of Midwives/Royal College of Obstetricians and Gynaecologists 2007; Royal College of Obstetricians and Gynaecologists 2008). Collaborative strategies to support maternity services have also transcended party political differences as evidenced by the All Party Parliamentary Group for Maternity (2010). The group receives expert advice on maternity issues from the Maternity Care Working Party which has wide representation from stakeholder organisations.

Moving policy into practice

Woven through these documents and initiatives, and a source of much debate, is the adoption of evidence-based care and its impact on appropriate use of interventions through pregnancy, labour and birth. However, despite a growing body of evidence demonstrating that CS operations are associated with risks for women and neonates (Deneux-Tharaux *et al.* 2006; Gray *et al.* 2007; Liu *et al.* 2007; Villar *et al.* 2007), rates continue to rise globally. In this case, the evidence base does not seem to be a powerful driver.

In 1985, against a background of concern about the rising CS rates, the World Health Organization (WHO) organised a consensus conference to explore the evidence around and drivers for caesarean section. It concluded that there were no additional health benefits associated with a CS rate above 10–15% (Thomas & Paranjothy 2001). Despite this, the rate of CS in England has continued to rise, doubling from 12% in 1990 to 24% in 2007. Indeed, rates are rising across the world. There is a growing body of clinical opinion that applying best practice in maternity care would result in achieving and maintaining CS rates below 20% (NHS Institute 2006a). Many maternity units are able to recognise what constitutes best practice, but experience difficulty in introducing and embedding change. The cultural shift that is required to realise a reduction in CS rates often goes unrecognised. Recommending a CS rate for units to aspire to, in the UK or elsewhere, is not therefore always helpful.

The NHS institute's *Delivering Quality and Value* programme

'High-volume care', part of the *Delivering Quality and Value* (DQV) programme at the NHS Institute, aims to discover how top-performing healthcare organisations in the NHS and elsewhere deliver the highest quality care with the best use of resources, and how to find effective ways of spreading that successful practice to other service providers (Baldwin *et al.* 2007).

Reflecting a collaborative method, the NHS Institute (2006b) stated that each programme should:

- be clinically led
- engage with a wide range of clinical and managerial professionals
- be co-produced with the NHS
- integrate with other NHS initiatives.

In the rest of this chapter, we will explore these elements through a case study of the NHS Institute's CS team.

In 2005, the Department of Health commissioned the NHS Institute's *Delivering Quality and Value* (DQV) programme to determine best practice in eight specific clinical pathways. These eight pathways were selected because they represented healthcare resource groups (HRGs) with high volumes of activity and where there was wide variation in clinical practice and performance across the country. The pathways included diverse clinical areas from adult mental health problems to cholecystectomy. Caesarean section was identified as one of these high-volume activities.

Focus on: Caesarean Section

In 2005, centrally collected statistics showed that over 135,000 caesarean operations had been performed in England (Hospital Episode Statistics 2006). The Department of Health further identified a variation in practice in postnatal management following caesarean section. Across England, the average postnatal stay varied from 3.5 days to 7 days, representing a significant difference in patterns of care for women and in resources related to bed usage.

Clinically led

Following the pattern established for all the DQV projects, the NHS Institute appointed a small team consisting of an NHS Institute associate to manage the project, a consultant obstetrician as clinical lead, an experienced health services improvement facilitator and a statistician. With the exception of the associate, the team members were all seconded part time to work on this project.

Having considered the Department of Health brief, the team decided that the most significant variation in clinical practice associated with CS was not the postnatal stay but the wide range of CS rates across maternity services in England. Statistics showed that some units maintained CS rates below 15% whilst others had rates in excess of 30%. Critically, this variation was not associated with improved perinatal outcomes. Less than half of the difference in rates could be ascribed to demography or to complexity of case mix, despite the fact that these characteristics are often quoted as the main reasons for differences in CS rates (Paranjothy *et al.* 2005).

Engagement with professionals

The team visited nine maternity services with a wide range of birth rates and different service configurations, in a variety of settings. We gathered information through interviews, observation in clinical areas, and by a review of documentation produced by each service. We carried out a series of semi-structured interviews with members of staff, which involved all professional disciplines at all levels, from the executive team to the support staff. We included those working on the wards and in clinics, and staff working wholly or principally in the community. Where maternity services had more than one physical base, we included at least one midwife-led unit in our visit. We spoke to women in antenatal clinics and postnatal wards to record their views on aspects of their maternity care. During observation periods we took the opportunity to talk informally to small groups of staff 'on the shop floor'.

The team made a baseline assessment of the demography of the population served, and gathered practical information on the organisational structure of the service, staffing numbers, configurations and working patterns. We examined the data collected by the unit. We rapidly determined that maternity data submitted centrally to the Department of Health were often an inaccurate reflection of true activity within individual maternity units. They were inadequate in identifying birth outcomes for local populations, as women having home births or using separate midwifery-led units were often omitted from the figures. Furthermore, conversations with individual members of staff within the same unit revealed wide variations in awareness of clinical outcomes, and large ranges of estimates of CS rates and normal birth rates. In fact, although four of the nine trusts visited had CS rates at or below 20%, the remaining five had a span of CS rates between 21% and 29% for their whole health communities.

Staff in those maternity services where CS rates were genuinely low identified a number of specific clinical practices and behaviours that they believed contributed to low CS rates, whilst providing a safe service. These 'high performers' were also able to look beyond the practical components of their systems to describe elements of the culture of their organisation. They considered high-quality leadership, multidisciplinary teamworking, communication, learning and governance to be fundamental to their success in maintaining their low CS rates. They described a shared vision for their service and demonstrated clarity of purpose that we did not observe in those units with high CS rates.

Co-production

Following the visits, we organised a 'co-production event', attended by multidisciplinary teams, including a senior midwife, a lead obstetrician and a senior manager from each of the services we had visited. We invited a further four high-performing maternity trusts to join the event. In a workshop setting, the participants worked collaboratively to review the accuracy and balance of the collated information our team had gathered. Having validated those practices and behaviours they considered to represent best practice, the group prioritised those characteristics they believed were most significant in maintaining low CS rates. We noted with interest that, although there were representatives of trusts with widely varying CS rates within the room, all the 'co-producers' were able to reach consensus on best practice, even when they were unable to achieve this themselves. The participants then discussed the key messages and underlying themes as they related to clinical practice.

Through this collaborative process, participants at the co-production event played a key role in shaping the future of this work. Their prioritisation provided the basis for the 'top ten' characteristics of high-performing services (Box 11.1).

Each of the statements in the 'top ten' reflects the importance of organisational culture in achieving a shared consensus and vision amongst members of the multidisciplinary team. In discussing the key underlying themes, the co-producers identified care pathways for groups of women for whom the application of best practice might be expected to have the greatest impact in achieving and maintaining low CS rates. These were:

- the care of women in their first pregnancy and labour
- the care of women who have had a previous CS birth
- the organisational culture of the maternity service.

Box 11.1 Top ten characteristics of high-performing services (NHS institute 2006a)

What are the characteristics of services aspiring to optimal care?

- We focus on keeping pregnancy and birth normal
- We are a real team – we understand and respect roles and expertise
- Our leaders are visible and vocal
- Our guidelines are evidence based and up to date
- We all practise to the same guidelines – no opting out
- We manage women's expectations and prepare them for the reality of labour
- We are proactive about VBAC, giving accurate information about risks and benefits
- If a caesarean is planned, the process is efficient and effective
- We get accurate, timely and relevant information on our performance
- We work closely with our users and stakeholders

To this, the NHS Institute team added a further group:

- the care of women having an elective CS.

The elective CS group was included partly in recognition of the original concern raised by the Department of Health on variation in postnatal stay, but also in response to observations that poor organisation of elective surgery was affecting the quality of the birth experience for the women themselves, and diverting resources from women in the other key groups above.

We took the key themes that emerged from the co-production event and organised them into pathways that represented the journey each group of women takes through maternity services, including the periods before and between pregnancies. We then took the best practice ideas identified and validated with the maternity services at the co-production event and aligned them with the four pathways listed above as the basis for our first publication, *Delivering Quality and Value. Focus On: Caesarean Section* (NHS Institute 2006a) The pathways were illustrated with brief case histories provided by units that had demonstrated examples of best practice.

The team then circulated the draft document to a wide group of stakeholders including academic bodies, professional colleges, policy bodies and user representatives for consultation. We invited their opinion on the content, the format and the language.

Following publication, the document was sent to all maternity services in England, so that the best practice identified could be shared with the wider NHS. Although the document was a useful source of information for maternity services aiming to reduce CS rates, a more practical approach was required for services to be able to implement these key characteristics of best practice.

Culture and collaboration

Best practice, despite evidence of effectiveness, is often not disseminated into clinical practice. Even when it is disseminated, it is often only partially adopted. For example, national guidance in 2001 recommended that the practice of routine electronic fetal monitoring in women with healthy pregnancies admitted in spontaneous labour should be discontinued (NICE 2001). However, it was evident from the visits and conversations we have had with midwives in England that this practice continues in some units. Most of these staff knew that this practice was no longer recommended, but either felt happier *doing what they had always done* or implied that *this was the way things are done around here*. This kind of behaviour is often reflective of organisational culture (Davies *et al.* 2000).

The presence and impact of organisationalZ culture were one of the key findings in our first phase of work in relation to reducing CS rates (NHS Institute 2006a). It is difficult to find a method which can address these issues without causing conflict. These findings are similar to the Ontario study (Ontario Women's Health Council 2000), which identified 12 critical success factors present in maternity units with low intervention rates. These included pride in a low CS rate, a 'culture' where birth is seen as a physiological event and commitment to one-to-one care in active labour. The work highlighted the importance of strong team leadership, effective multidisciplinary teams and access to professional skills. It is the shared experiences of the maternity team and the culture of the organisation which provide the stability and predictability that are crucial for meaningful collaborative work to occur (Weick 1995).

It was evident from our observations and discussions that, rather than just being given a list of best practice descriptors, maternity units needed practical assistance to address the issue of promoting normal birth and reducing CS rates.

We recognised that the methodology and design of such a toolkit should enable maternity staff to hold up a lens to their actions and behaviours. It should also facilitate staff in taking a fresh look at their service. This involved enabling staff to understand the impact of their actions and behaviours on clinical outcomes, and to make the link between their organisational culture and their intervention rates. It was also important that the toolkit should be highly user friendly and presented in a style and design that would promote open discussion between staff and service users.

In maternity services there are still instances where a lack of good communication and collaboration has a negative impact on maternal and infant well-being (Lewis 2007; O'Neill 2008). Recent quality and safety standards have acted as a powerful catalyst for maternity teams in the UK to embrace the concept of shared learning rather than separate training for professional groups. This is a strategy that has been shown to facilitate closer and more effective teamworking and collaboration (NHS Litigation Authority 2009; Royal College of Obstetricians and Gynaecologists 2008). As has been explored in Chapter 9, traditionally, midwives and obstetricians have been socialised and trained in competing paradigms, leading to different perspectives and thought processes (Davis-Floyd 2003). The divergence in views and values of professional groups often results in interprofessional conflict or a lack of consensus in how values are operationalised (Siddiqui 1996; Stapleton 1998). This lack of cohesion and understanding not only occurs between different professional groups, but is also evident amongst members of the same profession working together. Hunter (2004) reports how conflicting ideologies create the most disharmony and dissonance among colleagues. In her study, hospital-based midwives divided themselves into 'us and them' based on ideology. It is important that these differences in values and philosophies are openly discussed so that agreement can be reached and shared values and goals realised. This is the basis of good collaborative working (Stapleton 1998).

Pathways to Success – a self-improvement toolkit

In order to deliver the type of improvement toolkit that was needed, our first action was to reconfigure the CS team to embrace the multidisciplinary working pattern so strongly advocated by our 'high performers'. Two experienced midwives joined the team on part-time secondments in place of the service improvement facilitator. They acted as 'fresh eyes' in reviewing the information gathered in the production of the *Focus On* document, and they brought breadth and balance to the clinical perspective of the team.

The reconfigured team debated a change of emphasis from the objective of reducing CS rates to one of increasing normal birth rates. We were clear that successful service improvement in maternity care required commitment from all professional groups. In recent history, normal birth has often been regarded as the exclusive domain of the midwife, and the care of women with complications as that of the obstetrician. To reconcile these positions and achieve a balanced approach, we named the next phase of our work *Pathways to Success: Focus on Normal Birth and Reducing Caesarean Section Rates.*

Our challenge was to transform the information underpinning the *Focus On: Caesarean Section* best practice document into a practical toolkit that maternity teams could use to understand their processes and behaviours. We also wanted them to engage in debate about how these might impact on their clinical outcomes, and to provide tried and tested tools and innovative ideas to help them make sustainable changes in their maternity services.

We decided to build on the structure of the four key pathways set out above. Elements of best practice were arranged in the sequence of a woman's journey though maternity care. We then used the evidence gathered from our original observations and interviews. We augmented these with specific examples provided during the co-production and consultation processes, as concrete examples of existing practice. The examples were chosen to reflect not only systems and processes in use in maternity services, but also the attitudes and behaviours of those delivering care. The team then integrated the associated examples with the pathways to form a 'maturity matrix' so that the woman's journey is displayed on the vertical axis of the grid and the examples of processes and behaviours are displayed from left to right progressively representing services with lower CS rates (Figure 11.1).

The concept of a maturity matrix was developed in the context of process improvements in information technology (Crosby 1979). The progression to maturity allows individuals or teams to establish a baseline and to work through a staged process towards the optimal position, with reference to a particular characteristic, process or system. It has been applied in other spheres and there is evidence of its successful application in healthcare (National Patient Safety Agency 2006). In our maturity matrix, the characteristics form the steps on the woman's journey through each pathway. The staged process takes maternity units through an improvement journey towards the declared objective, that of promoting normal birth and reducing CS rates.

All the material used to populate the matrix came from information provided by or practices we observed in maternity services in England. Not all the practices attributed to the high performers follow evidence-based care, usually because the evidence in this area is not yet available. In other instances, evidence has become available during the lifetime of the project. The ability to see what has been 'tried and tested' in high-performing organisations is also useful in encouraging debate around what could or should be possible in other maternity services.

The CS team recognised the importance of the cultural issues underlying all aspects of maternity care. High performers placed great

Postnatal care

Inter-pregnancy

Antenatal care

Labour and birth

Antenatal

Women choose VBAC when clinically appropriate	"Once a section always a section- the woman expects an operation." Midwives lack confidence and experience in VBAC	There is difference of opinion between clinicians. Midwives and women are confused about plans of care.	Clinician's support VBAC in some cases but decisions must be make by a senior doctor, women are not seen untill 36 weeks in case other problems occur affecting delivery plans.	There is a designated appointment in early pregnancy to discuss VBAC. Other professionals respect the decision made.	Women and professionals are well informed about VBAC. Women arrive at their booking appointment confident about VBAC. Choices are confirmed early in pregnancy.
Midwives are skilled in risk assessment and confident in advising women about VBAC	Midwives actively avoid discussing mode of delivery after previous section.	Midwives feel empowered to discuss mode of delivery but are not allowed to make the final decision.	Midwives are able to discuss mode of birth with women but the decision for VBAC can only be made after discussion with consultant midwife or obstetrician.	All midwives are able to discuss and agree mode of birth with women. Women are cared for by midwives but have a named consultant.	All midwives are able to discuss and agree mode of birth and offer midwifery-led care without medical involvement.
We are committed to the philosophy of facilitating a normal birth with women who have experienced a CS	Women have already made their minds up when they book. If they ask for CS we accept their choice. Staff avoid discussing mode of delivery in early pregnancy.	If a woman asks for CS we accept her choice after telling her about the relative risks and benefits of CS and VBAC.	If women ask for CS with no clear indication we go through the motions of asking for a second opinion before we say yes.	Dedicated multidisciplinary VBAC clinic provides information and support to those undecided about mode of birth.	All staff are able to discuss the benefits of VBAC. The possibility of VBAC is explored with all women.
Antenatal care is unaffected by previous CS	Following CS, this is automatically a high risk pregnancy and is managed by obstetricians.	These women may be at greater antenatal risk so should be seen in hospital as well as in the community.	All women with previous CS must be seen at least once by the obstetrician to confirm mode of delivery.	Women receive midwife-led care but are routinely offered an appointment with the obstetrician during their pregnancy.	Women who have had a previous CS receive midwife-led antenatal care. The referral criteria are identical with those for other pregnant women.

Figure 11.1 Example from the *Pathway for care for women who have had a previous CS.* Copyright NHS Institute for Innovation and Improvement (2007), all rights reserved.

emphasis on good interdisciplinary working, leadership and communication. We therefore devised a framework in which the toolkit maturity matrices could be used to promote improvements in these aspects as well as making changes in processes and systems.

Having devised the maturity matrix that underpins the toolkit, we carried out a consultation process with the original contributors and with the representative bodies that commented on the *Focus On: Caesarean Section* document, and incorporated their suggestions. The draft toolkit was also circulated for comment and discussion to user organisations including the National Childbirth Trust, the Birth Trauma Association and some Maternity Service Liaison Committee (MSLC) chairs. We were particularly interested in their comments on the appropriateness of the language within the toolkit. We then began a programme of pilots, in which we facilitated workshops within individual maternity services to test the appropriateness of the pathway format. This allowed us to gain feedback on the experience of using the toolkit.

The toolkit was designed to be used in the context of multidisciplinary workshops, where people from all professional groups, and at all levels in the organisation, could work together on an improvement journey. This format encourages all professional groups to identify a shared vision. The vision then generates a shared responsibility for changing those systems and behaviours that often impact on promoting normality. In this way, change is owned by all participants, rather than being the 'job' or 'role' of one professional group. The benefit of having involvement from service users at these workshops is highlighted as good practice in the toolkit. Their contribution is invaluable in providing an alternative view to that of the professional groups.

We conducted workshops using the pathway matrices in the toolkit with 12 maternity services. In the majority of cases, we provided the facilitation for the process. On two occasions, we were observers when the host unit conducted its own workshop. At each of these pilot workshops, we asked participants to concentrate on a chosen pathway (first pregnancy and labour, vaginal birth after caesarean (VBAC), elective caesarean or organisational). Through discussion and debate, we asked them to establish where their service currently sat on the maturity matrix. At all these pilot sites, the pathways enabled participants to highlight differences in perceptions amongst staff who worked together but nonetheless held differing views and ideas which they had not previously discussed together. These differences in perception were sometimes due to the physical separation of teams, as in the case of hospital midwives and community midwives. Sometimes it was a hierarchical separation, based on level of seniority. In each case, the debate highlighted a lack of knowledge and understanding of each other's roles.

> *Absolutely great to discuss our service with a mix of totally relevant people. Makes me realise how isolated I usually am day to day.*
>
> (Midwife, North Bristol)

We also noted that professionals often believed that the way they practise is the same as everyone else, and that they were unaware of the variation from practitioner to practitioner. We frequently heard comments from medical registrars that 'I have always debriefed my caesarean section women on the postnatal ward before they go home' and, from midwives, that 'I always encourage women to try for a normal birth after a previous CS'. The discovery that not everyone was practising to the same standards often came as a great surprise to the individuals concerned. The process of following the pathway highlighted to midwives and obstetricians not only the inconsistencies in practice and beliefs but also their limited insight into the complete journey that women took through their service. They became aware that they tended to concentrate on their own involvement and were not conscious of how the rest of the system behaved.

We received positive evaluations from all the pilot sites, citing particularly the value of the approach in fostering open discussion and debate amongst staff with a wide range of roles and experiences.

> *Everyone who took part in the workshop found it a useful exercise, both in terms of thinking about where we were as a directorate in relation to the examples quoted, and in terms of the multidisciplinary communication and learning that happened as a consequence.*
>
> (Head of Midwifery, East Sussex)

The CS team made a conscious choice to use the maturity matrix format to display the pathways because it gave participants the permission they needed to explore the ideas and behaviours that exist in their organisation, however implicit or explicit they appear. This phenomenon is sometimes referred to as the 'elephant in the room'. It describes how people are often willing to ignore the presence of obvious behaviours, processes and important topics because initiating this discussion is too uncomfortable. Direct observation of discussion groups and feedback from participants consistently confirmed that the workshop environment was sufficiently supportive to allow them to debate issues they would hesitate to raise in their normal working environment.

> *Very interesting to hear views from all disciplines, particularly consultants who I rarely have the opportunity to hear from. Lots of information and real inside view of what the service thinks of itself as opposed to what we the users think of it.*
>
> (Service user, West Suffolk)

The successful piloting of the pathways in the multidisciplinary workshops enabled the team to refine the marketing of the toolkit and add a CD-ROM containing a wide range of tools to help maternity units make improvements in their services. We also produced detailed guidance on facilitation of the workshops to assist multidisciplinary maternity teams through the assessment and improvement process. The finished toolkit was launched as a self-directed, self-contained package that could be taken up and used by any maternity unit. It was published in 2007 as *Pathways to Success: A Self-Improvement Toolkit: Focus On Normal Birth And Reducing CS Rates* (NHS Institute 2007).

Discussion

Collaboration can be defined simply as two or more people coming together to discuss a common problem (Lockhart-Wood 2000). As has been noted in Chapter 9, collaboration in healthcare can take different forms. It can occur between staff groups, between organisations, and between professionals and patients. The focus tends to be the needs of the patient, with negotiations resulting in a plan of care (Henneman *et al.* 1995; Lockhart-Wood 2000). Effective collaboration, however, does not simply exist due to the close proximity of professionals literally working together to provide care. It requires time and conscious effort. Evans (1994, p.22) describes a dynamic relationship that requires respect between professionals as 'a synergistic alliance that maximises the contribution of each participant, resulting in action that is greater than the sum of individual works'.

Collaborative working requires equity in terms of professional status and roles – something which can conflict with the hierarchical model of working that is standard in many formal healthcare settings.

Approaches such as the Midwifery Partnership Model (Guilliland & Pairman 1995) extend the concept of equity beyond professional boundaries. Derived from observational research of midwifery practice in New Zealand, this theory proposes an approach where the midwife and woman hold equal power in their relationship with each other, whilst having different knowledge and expertise. The woman is seen to have a particular kind of experiential expertise in childbirth. The partnership develops from genuine collaboration towards shared meaning through mutual understanding (Guilliland & Pairman 1995). In this model, collaboration with women is central to understanding childbirth and, ultimately, women's experience of childbirth and how to improve that experience. From a similar philosophical position, Benbow *et al.* (1997) suggest that the maternity service needs to focus on breaking down professional barriers to establish collaboration and co-operation among professions, and a team approach which recognises the woman as a team member.

As discussed in Chapter 9, the terms 'interdisciplinary', 'multiprofessional' and 'multidisciplinary' are used interchangeably in the literature (Payne 2000; Leathard 2003). In clinical practice, the term 'collaboration' is commonly used yet poorly understood, and often inappropriately applied (Henneman *et al.* 1995). On occasions, it is applied to denote the physical presence of different professionals, rather than purposive engagement in an interactive process.

For effective collaboration to take place, Keleher (1998) notes that the following characteristics are essential: mutual trust and respect; valuing each other's perspectives; equality and shared responsibility; and professional competence. Henneman *et al.* (1995) use the terms 'participation', 'autonomy' and 'interdependence' as critical to effective collaboration. Communication is also cited as key (Stapleton 1998).

Using the toolkit to facilitate collaborative working and reduce CS rates

Achieving effective collaboration at local level is not always easy. Lack of time and pressure of work are often disabling factors. In the maternity care context, operational issues also act as barriers. These include shift times, which result in midwives and obstetricians starting at different times of the day, and separate handovers for the different professional groups, making discussion and interaction difficult.

Effective collaboration is a dynamic process that demands certain characteristics in order to be successful. The practical nature of the *Pathways to Success* toolkit requires the multidisciplinary team to discuss and explore their individual opinions and share differences in perception in order to explore and agree new ways of working. Creating an appropriate environment for professionals to be able to discuss and debate openly such differences and acknowledge diversity of opinions is crucial. Effective maternity care does not consist only of delivering validated forms of care with expertise. Care delivery must take into account social relationships, social and psychological processes, and concepts such as hierarchy, autonomy, status, power, vested interests and charisma (MacIntyre & Porter 1989). The maturity matrix methodology of the toolkit, which captures actions and behaviours that exist in maternity services across England, encourages participants to make an open and honest self-assessment of their own current organisational and clinical systems.

> *The pathways support issues that are not often discussed or even acknowledged within an organisation. The culture of your organisation is paramount in reducing CS rates.*
>
> (Maternity and Gynaecology Manager)

The maturity matrices deliberately present practices that are often not talked about but which exist behind closed doors. By making visible in the narrative of the matrix those things not often even spoken about, 'It is almost as if permission is given to make negative comments where appropriate, as this can be done by using the phrases listed' (Gulati 2007). Having seen that certain practices exist 'elsewhere', it seems to be easier to acknowledge them in one's own service. This is an important part of understanding the genuine starting point, from which everyone can agree the next steps forward. From all the workshops we observed or facilitated, evaluations have described the workshop as 'a positive experience', the vast majority of respondents have reported that the workshop made them reflect differently on the care they give, and that it highlighted areas for improvement to focus on.

> *Good platform to know where we are and differences in opinion among*
> *multidisciplinary team so it is easier to focus on what we need to do.*
> (Obstetrician)

Respondents also reported that they were able to express their opinions, felt they had gained more of a shared vision, and believed that attending the workshop would make a difference to how they practised. The fact that these discussions have taken place between and across professional and lay groups makes them all the more powerful as a starting point for collaborative service transformation. If the culture of an organisation is its internalised values, beliefs and aspirations, then good quality is dependent on these factors (Buchanan *et al.* 2007). The development work around the CS initiative seems to encourage this kind of quality, by testing and reorientating the local culture.

> *'Excellent venue for enabling lively debate. Definitely challenges conven-*
> *tional dogma.* (Community midwife)

> *Enabled good multidisciplinary approach and discussion, good to have open*
> *discussion and relook at culture, practice and habits in the unit.* (Midwife)

An important aspect of the workshops is the social interaction that takes place among group members. This is similar to the collaborative learning models that Schwartz (1999) describes. These models suggest a move from assimilation to construction, whereby members create new understandings based on the discussions they have had.

> *Having tried to improve normality and normal birth environment for so*
> *long using the multidisciplinary situation, today has been so positive.*
> (Midwife)

One element that is key to promoting normal birth and reducing CS is the awareness that these two elements are complementary aspects of the same objective of good-quality maternity care. They are not distinguished by professional boundaries and are therefore 'everybody's business'. Some authors go so far as to suggest that 'without the positive involvement and engagement of all clinicians . . . attempts at large-scale change are doomed' (Ham & Dickinson 2008).

Leadership versus leaders in a collaborative model

The toolkit describes the need for a structured group to lead the self-improvement process, and recommends developing a small core team of people who own and guide the process rather than appointing individuals as leaders. This should include midwives and obstetricians who are enthusiasts for the project and ideally have special skills, or those who hold positions of responsibility or influence in their service (NHS Institute 2007). Their role is more closely aligned to a facilitation role, thus 'creating the conditions to release potential energy' (Bate 1994, p.245). The core team should create an environment which can 'encourage and support the individual development of leadership skills' (Outhwaite 2003).

The concept of *shared leadership* discussed in Chapter 1 of this volume is relevant to the issues debated in this chapter. In this case, 'leadership occurs at every level and is not the sole responsibility of individuals at the top of their organisation' (NHS Institute/Academy of Medical Royal Colleges 2008). As the NHS Institute (2007) notes: 'We are all potential leaders. We champion our service and all work to make it better'.

Spread and adopt strategies for sustainable change

Recent healthcare improvement literature estimates that 15–20% of NHS staff are engaged in quality improvement work in order to try and meet the goals as set out in *The NHS Plan* (NHS Institute 2009c). It is also estimated that achievement of these goals may require 80% or 100% of staff engagement (NHS Institute 2009c). Spread and Adopt strategies are one of the techniques used to encourage this more widespread buy-in. They acknowledge that the spread of good practice is closely linked to how communication functions within a social system (Fraser 2001). New ideas, innovations and practices are usually promulgated by the few (Fraser 2007). Rogers' work on the diffusion of innovation described the rate at which an innovation could be adopted, with a 'tipping point' marking the point at which a critical mass of adopters is achieved. He described diffusion as a process by which innovation is communicated among members in a social system. In this analysis, the tipping point denotes the development of a collective consciousness (Rogers 2003).

Spread and Adopt strategies are generally regarded as 'top-down' hierarchical models driven by those with power and influence. Although our work was commissioned by the Department of Health, the best practice promoted in the *Pathways to Success* toolkit was derived from collaborative working with maternity teams at grass-roots level.

Good Spread and Adopt processes are only half the story. The recipients of the information need to be open to the possibility of change. In addition, the degree to which individuals engage in innovation is strongly influenced by their perception of the need to change (Fraser 2001, 2007). When like-thinking individuals join together in a common recognition of the need to change their world, the impetus is energised and gains momentum. There has been increasing interest in whether social movement theory could provide useful insight into large-scale systems change (Bate *et al.* 2005). The concept of the collective consciousness is an inherent part of social movement theory. Social movements have been described as 'involving collective action by individuals who have voluntarily come together around a common cause; they often involve radical action and protest, which may lead to conflict with accepted norms and "ways of doing" things' (Bate *et al.* 2005, p.12.) Social movement theory problematises the ways in which people live their lives, and offers the potential for changes in habits of thought, action and interpretation (Crossley 2002). Engagement with specific social movements can play an important part in consciousness raising towards collective action (Bate *et al.* 2005).

The toolkit is a vehicle for the spread and adoption of maternity improvements designed to promote normal birth and reduce CS rates. The methodology underpinning the maturity matrices allows participants in maternity services to reach a collective view about their current practices and for them to identify any shared dissatisfaction with the status quo.

From collaborative working within maternity units to collaborative working amongst maternity services

The publication of *Pathways to Success* created considerable interest within maternity services. The NHS Institute received many requests from units for help in implementing the toolkit locally. In response to this, a Spread and Adopt strategy was implemented by the CS team to provide tailored support to 20 maternity units. Furthermore, in order to support more units in using the toolkit and to spread new ways of working to promote normality and reduce CS rates, the team conducted network events with each of the ten SHAs in England. The intention was to generate a network of people talking about the possibility for change within maternity services, and to use these events to inform, debate and build on the original work by collaborating with a wider network of people. It also provided an invaluable opportunity for regional groups to learn about different practices and ideas from neighbouring hospitals.

Networks have been described as a 'social pursuit with purpose' (DH 2006) and can be a powerful lever for change (Pettigrew *et al*. 1992). They are said to provide collaborative advantage (DH 2006). This is because innovation is a social interactive process, rather than an individual creative one (Hargreaves 2004). When groups of people come together with common interests and passions, they share and learn together (DH 2006).

Many organisations commented in their evaluation that it was good to hear about other practices and to network with colleagues. During many of the network events, we encouraged organisations to explore the highlights and challenges within their service. During this activity, it became apparent that maternity units were at different stages in their improvement journeys. Often, *the answer was in the room*. Bevan *et al*. (2008) believe that moving from a good to a great service involves understanding that many of the answers lie within. This means engaging front-line staff much more fully than before in service transformation (Bevan *et al*. 2008).

Developing local solutions

We are often asked 'Can you tell us what is working elsewhere?'. Part of our work has involved sharing ideas from other units, in order to spread good practice. There are some key innovations that the high performers have found helpful. These have been disseminated to other units that have, in their turn, benefited from them (Box 11.2).

We also stress that developing an in-house (local) solution is vital. The 'high performers' who provided the original best practices in the toolkit had characteristics that allowed them to develop their services quickly and adapt to changing situations. In terms of their ability to embrace and adopt new ideas, they might be what Rogers (2003) called 'innovators' and other authors have called 'enthusiasts' (Fraser 2007). Fraser describes the characteristics of enthusiasts as forward-looking and able to demonstrate initiative, excitement and creativity (Fraser 2007). She suggests that they operate outside the 'norm' and she questions whether it is reasonable to expect the large majority of people to adopt a solution developed outside the norm (Fraser 2007).

Fraser also cautions against the one-size-fits-all solution to an issue, as it limits diversity (Fraser 2007), and diversity is important to sustainability. Bevan *et al*. (2008) indicate that a better balance needs to be struck between competition and collaboration. While they acknowledge that competition can drive up standards, it can also become a barrier to collaboration. In contrast, Fraser argues that creating a marketplace

---

Box 11.2   Key innovations in high-performing units (NHS institute 2007)

Twenty four-hour multidisciplinary case review

There is a multidisciplinary review of care daily; all emergency CS as well as births with a positive outcome are discussed. There is an open and honest 'no blame' culture.

Effective external cephalic version (ECV) pathway for babies presenting by the breech

All staff feel confident to discuss ECV, including benefits and risks. Each woman receives written information. There is a high uptake of ECV.

Letter to all women following an emergency CS

Doctors and midwives discuss the birth events with each woman and document the discussion and outcomes in the records. Women receive written information about the reasons for their CS. This letter is copied to the GP and community midwife.

Twenty four-hour triage away from labour ward

The labour ward is kept free for labouring women. Women are assessed prior to arriving on the labour ward either at home or through the triage system.

Appropriate utilisation of staff

Women receive one-to-one support in labour from a midwife. The skill mix is used innovatively to enable midwives to do this. The personnel and skill mix for theatre are organised to reduce impact on management on labouring women.

---

where there is competition is important, as participants in the market-place can make choices and continue to adapt and grow (Fraser 2007). She states that an organisation may take on and promote a specific model, but this may be to the detriment of diversity and other possibilities (Fraser 2007). As an alternative, she suggests that multiple strategies and feedback systems are needed to encourage innovation. During our network events, we have found that all organisations are happy to share ideas. The diversity evident in this networking enables participants to go beyond the good practice highlighted within the toolkit to create new visions and possibilities.

As Fraser states, spread is about communication: 'we need to involve others . . . raise awareness of the issues and ownership of the solutions' (Fraser 2007, p.14). Using the toolkit methodology to explore a starting position, to arrive at a collective aspiration for the future of a service, and to understand the incremental steps that may be required along the way can support large-scale change required to influence organisational culture within maternity services. As Fraser states, it is necessary 'to retain all your existing knowledge and build on it' (2007, p.43). Research on large-scale change shows that if services are to improve dramatically, it will be through the engaged improvement efforts of front-line and managerial staff who do the work (Bevan *et al.* 2008). Whilst bringing in 'outside' change experts and consultancies can add momentum, new perspective and skills in the short term, it is the 'inside' change, the capability of the system (and the people within it) to change that will create the sustainable improvements (Bevan *et al.* 2008).

Conclusion

The *Pathways to Success* toolkit has been developed by the NHS Institute for Innovation and Improvement to address the issue of rising CS rates in England. The toolkit design reflects the fact that effective maternity care is not merely the physical delivery of appropriate, safe care but also a dynamic interaction that takes place within a social context (MacIntyre & Porter 1989).

The toolkit design has evolved through collaborative working with a range of maternity units and considerable dialogue from all levels of staff providing maternity care, as well as from service users and other stakeholders. Rather than offering formal instruction or a collation of research or best practice, it has been designed as a practical self-improvement tool for use by the multidisciplinary team.

The toolkit enables multidisciplinary groups working together to share their differences in perception. It allows the variation in practices between clinicians to be highlighted. The effect of this on the woman's journey through the maternity service can be mapped. Evidence from social sciences suggests that the inclusion of a range of perspectives may complement improvement thinking and practice. Change can be driven and sustained through engaging with core values of individuals, and mobilising their own internal energies and drivers for change (NHS Institute 2009c). In this way, shared understanding is promoted, leading to alteration in collective behaviours and to collective action (McAdam 1986).

The *Pathways to Success: A Self-Improvement Toolkit: Focus On Normal Birth And Reducing CS Rates* is a practical toolkit for engaging maternity staff and women in working towards a common goal and shared vision. It provides a platform for improved collaborative working. Crucially, it provides the philosophical space in which maternity services can address the often subliminal and difficult aspects of organisational culture, which have an impact on CS rates and the provision of maternity care as a whole.

References

All Party Parliamentary Group for Maternity (2010) *Who We Are*. www .appg–maternity.org.uk/2.html (accessed June, 2010).

Baldwin J, Brodrick A, Mason N, Cowley S (2007) A clear focus: caesareans in the spotlight. *Practising Midwife* 10(3): 28–31.

Bate P (1994) *Strategies for Cultural Change*. Oxford, Butterworth.

Bate P, Bevan H, Robert G (2005) *Towards A Million Change Agents. A Review of the Social Movement Literature: Implications for Large Scale Change in the NHS*. London, NHS Modernisation Agency.

Benbow A, Semple D, Maresh M (1997) *Effective Procedures in Maternity Care Suitable for Audit*. London, Royal College of Obstetricians and Gynaecologists Press.

Bevan H, Ham C, Plsek P (2008) The next leg of the journey: how do we make *High Quality Care for All a reality?* Coventry, NHS Institute for Innovation and Improvement.

Buchanan DA, Fitzgerald L, Ketley D (2007) *The Sustainability and Spread of Organizational Change: Modernizing Healthcare*. London, Routledge.

Crosby P (1979) *Quality is Free: The Art of Making Quality Certain*. London, McGraw-Hill.

Crossley N (2002) *Making Sense of Social Movements*. Buckingham, Open University Press.

Davies H, McNutley S, Mannion R (2000) Organisational culture and quality of health care. *Quality in Health Care* 9:111–19.

Davis-Floyd R.E. (2003) *Birth as an American Rite of Passage*. Berkeley, CA, University of California Press.

Deneux-Tharaux C, Carmona E, Bouvier-Colle M, Breart G (2006) Postpartum maternal mortality and Caesarean delivery. *Obstetrics and Gynecology* 108: 541–8.

Department of Health (1993) *Changing Childbirth: Report of the Expert Maternity Group*. London, HMSO.

Department of Health (2000) *The NHS Plan: A Plan for Investment, A Plan for Reform*. London, Stationery Office.

Department of Health (2006) *Designing Networks for Collaborative Advantage: Practice Based Evidence on How to Set Up Networks to Improve Partnership Working and Achieve Positive Outcomes*. London, Care Service Improvement Partnership.

Department of Health (2007a) *Our NHS, Our Future: The Next Stage Review, Interim Report*. London, Department of Health.

Department of Health (2007b) *Maternity Matters: Choice, Access and Continuity of Care in a Safe Service*. London, Department of Health.

Department of Health (2008) *High Quality Care for All: NHS Next Stage Review Final Report*. London, Department of Health.

Department of Health/NHS Finance, Performance and Operations (2008) *The Operating Framework for 2009/10 for the NHS in England*. London, Department of Health.

Evans J (1994) The role of the nurse manager in creating an environment for collaborative practice. *Holistic Nursing Practice* 8: 22–31.

Fraser SW (2001) *When Spread Slows Down*. Improvement Bulletin Number 12. www.sfassociates.biz/ (accessed June, 2010).

Fraser SW (2007) Undressing the Elephant. Why Good Practice Does Not Spread In Healthcare. Available from www.lulu.com (accessed June, 2010).

Gray R, Quigley M, Hockley C, Kurinczuk J, Goldacre M, Brocklehurst P (2007) Caesarean delivery and risk of stillbirth in subsequent pregnancy: a retrospective cohort study in an English population. *British Journal of Obstetrics and Gynaecology* 114(3): 264–70.

Guilliland K, Pairman S (1995) *The Midwifery Partnership: A Model for Practice*. Monograph series 95/1, Department of Nursing and Midwifery. Wellington, New Zealand, Victoria University of Wellington.

Gulati C (2007) An opportunity not to be missed: the new self-improvement toolkit for maternity units. *NCT Bulletin*, May.

Ham C, Dickinson H (2008) *Engaging Doctors in Leadership: What Can We Learn From International Experience And Research Evidence?* Coventry, NHS Institute for Innovation and Improvement.

Hargreaves D (2004) Networks, knowledge and innovation. In McCarthy H, Miller P, Skidmore P (eds) *Network Logic: Who Governs in an Interconnected World?* London, Demos.

Henneman EA, Lee JL, Cohen JI (1995) Collaboration: a concept analysis. *Journal of Advanced Nursing* 21: 103–9.

House of Commons (2007) Statement to the House of Commons by Rt Hon Alan Johnson MP, Secretary of State for Health, 4 July, on the Darzi review of the NHS. www.dh.gov.uk/en/MediaCentre/Speeches/DH_076534

Hospital Episode Statistics (2006) NHS National Maternity Statistics England 2005-6. Health and Social Care Information Centre. www.ic.nhs.uk/webfiles/publications/maternity0506/NHSMaternityStatsEngland200506_fullpublication%20V3.pdf (accessed June, 2010).

Hunter B (2004) Conflicting ideologies as a source of emotion work in midwifery. *Midwifery* 20: 261–72.

Keleher K (1998) Collaboration: characteristics, barriers and implications for midwifery. *Journal of Nurse-Midwifery* 43(1): 8–11.

Leathard A (2003) *Interprofessional Collaboration*. London, Brunner-Routledge.

Lewis G (ed) (2007) *Saving Mothers' Lives: Reviewing Maternal Deaths to Make Motherhood Safer –2003–2005*. The Seventh Report on Confidential Enquiries into Maternal Deaths in the United Kingdom. London, Confidential Enquiry into Maternal and Child Health.

Liu T, Chen C, Tsai Y (2007) Taiwan's high rate of Caesarean births: impacts of National Health Insurance and fetal gender preferences. *Birth* 34(2): 115–22.

Lockhart-Wood K (2000) Collaboration between nurses and doctors in clinical practice. *British Journal of Nursing* 9(5): 276–80.

MacIntyre S, Porter M (1989) Prospects and problems in promoting effective care at the local level. In Chalmers I, Enkin M, Keirse MJNC (eds) *Effective Care in Pregnancy and Childbirth*. Oxford, Oxford University Press.

McAdam D (1986) Recruitment to high risk activism: the case of freedom summer. *American Journal of Sociology* 2: 64–90.

National Childbirth Trust/Royal College of Midwives/Royal College of Obstetricians and Gynaecologists (2007) *Making Normal Birth a Reality: Consensus Statement from the Maternity Care Working Party*. London, National Childbirth Trust.

National Institute for Clinical Excellence (2001) *Electronic Fetal Monitoring: The Use and Interpretation of Cardiotography in Intrapartum Fetal Surveillance*. Inherited clinical guideline C. London, National Institute for Clinical Excellence.

National Institute for Clinical Excellence (2007) *Intrapartum Care Guideline*. London, National Institute for Clinical Excellence.

National Patient Safety Agency (2006) *Manchester Patient Safety Framework (MaPSaF) Facilitator Guidance*. Manchester, University of Manchester.

NHS Institute for Innovation and Improvement (2006a) *Delivering Quality and Value. Focus On: Caesarean Section*. Coventry, NHS Institute for Innovation and Improvement.

NHS Institute for Innovation and Improvement (2006b) *DQV– An Introduction*. NHS Institute internal document. Coventry, NHS Institute for Innovation and Improvement.

NHS Institute for Innovation and Improvement (2007) *Pathways to Success: A Self-Improvement Toolkit: Focus On Normal Birth And Reducing CS Rates*. Coventry, NHS Institute for Innovation and Improvement.

NHS Institute for Innovation and Improvement (2009a) www.institute.nhs.uk.

NHS Institute for Innovation and Improvement (2009b) *It's How We Do Things Around Here: An Introduction to the NHS Institute's Work Process*. www.institute.nhs.uk/images/documents/About_US/work%20process%20summary%20doc.pdf (accessed June, 2010).

NHS Institute for Innovation and Improvement (2009c) *The Power of One, The Power of Many: Bringing Social Movement Thinking to Health And Healthcare Improvement*. Coventry, NHS Institute for Innovation and Improvement. www.institute.nhs.uk/building_capability/new_model_for_transforming_the_nhs/the_power_of_one_the_power_of_many.html (accessed June, 2010).

NHS Institute for Innovation and Improvement and the Academy of Medical Royal Colleges (2008) *Engaging Doctors: Can Doctors Influence Organisational Performance?* Coventry, NHS Institute for Innovation and Improvement.

NHS Litigation Authority (2009) *Clinical Negligence Scheme for Trusts. Maternity Clinical Risk Management Standards. Version 2 2009/10*. London, NHS Litigation Authority.

O'Neill O (2008) *Safe Births: Everybody's Business*. London, King's Fund.

Ontario Women's Health Council (2000) *Attaining and Maintaining Best Practices in the Use of Caesarean Sections*. Toronto, Caesarean Section Working Group.

Outhwaite S (2003) The importance of leadership in an integrated team. *Journal of Nursing Management* 11:371–6.

Paranjothy S, Frost C, Thomas J (2005) How much variation in CS rates can be explained by case mix differences? *British Journal of Obstetrics and Gynaecology* 112:658–66.

Payne M (2000) *Team Work in Multi-Professional Care*. London, Palgrave.

Pettigrew A, Ferlie E, McKee L (1992) *Shaping Strategic Change*. London, Sage Publications.

Rogers E (2003) *Diffusion of Innovation*, 5th edn.New York, Free Press.

Royal College of Obstetricians and Gynaecologists (2008) *Standards for Maternity Care: Report of a Working Party*. London, Royal College of Obstetricians and Gynaecologists Press.

Schwartz DL (1999) The productive agency that drives collaborative learning. In Dillenbourg P,(ed) *Collaborative Learning: Cognitive and Computional Approaches*. Amsterdam, Pergamon.

Siddiqui J (1996) Midwifery values: part 1. *British Journal of Midwifery* 42: 87–9.

Stapleton SR (1998) Making collaborative practice work. *Journal of Nurse-Midwifery* 43(1): 12–18.

Thomas J, Paranjothy S (2001) The National Sentinel Caesarean Section Audit Report. London, Royal College of Obstetricians and Gynaecologists Press, London.

Villar J, Carroli G, Zavaleta, N *et al.* (2007) Maternal and neonatal risks and benefits associated with Caesarean delivery: multicentre prospective study. *British Medical Journal* 335(7628): 1025.

Weick KE (1995) *Sensemaking in Organizations*. London, Sage Publications.

Chapter 12
Bringing It All Together

Soo Downe, Louise Simpson and Sheena Byrom

The motivation for this book arose from personal experience, anecdote, storytelling and a series of formal research studies. All of us have a strong belief in the powerful effect of positive and engaged staff on optimal maternity care. All of us have worked with charismatic and dynamic colleagues. As a respondent in one of our studies commented of a 'good' leader she knew, 'she sort of shines' (Byrom & Downe 2010). This may imply that these individuals were held apart from the rest of the staff, in senior roles and in strategic positions. On the contrary, as some of the examples in the case studies in the book illustrate, people who stand out are often those who are not in formal leadership positions. They are those who work with mutual respect and trust with others in their group, and who are keen to maximise the well-being of the women they care for, and the staff they work with.

There are, however, influential people who are in formal leadership positions. Many of the authors of the chapters presenting case studies are in these roles. These individuals are prime examples of those who demonstrate expertise, transformational leadership and collaborative approaches. They are also those who take calculated risks at the boundaries of normally acceptable practice. This includes people like Fen Cheung, who has constructively challenged the highly technocratic maternity care norms of a whole country by creating a birth centre in China where, in some hospitals, caesarean section rates have reached 100%. It also includes Ann Davenport, who has had the humility to learn from traditional midwives. These accounts illustrate the fact that progression towards the best possible quality care depends on being 'open' and on 'sharing', in the words of Fen Cheung and Anita Fleming. These

Essential Midwifery Practice: Leadership, Expertise and Collaborative Working,
first edition. Edited by Soo Downe, Sheena Byrom and Louise Simpson
Published 2011 by Blackwell Publishing Ltd.
© 2011 Blackwell Publishing Ltd.

characteristics are relevant to all of the three areas that this book encompasses.

Leadership

There is a plethora of literature on the subject of leadership. Leadership styles, traits, characteristics and philosophies have interested management gurus and world leaders alike, and researchers have pursued the ultimate models for leadership as the route to organisational success. Leadership theory has been applied to nursing in the pursuit to improve standards of patient care and related health outcomes.

Midwifery leadership has received less attention than nursing leadership in terms of research and expert opinion, but as outlined in the leadership chapter of this book, it is an increasingly debated topic, with significant investment in the development of midwifery leaders (International Congress of Midwives 2010; Royal College of Midwives 2010). Midwifery leaders are required to do more than manage a service; there are midwifery leaders developing practice, managing risk, promoting normal birth and improving public health (Osbourne 2004). There are midwives working as professors of midwifery, and midwives working strategically to influence policy, national and international directives. In addition, there are midwives who quietly support, nurture and 'lead' women throughout pregnancy and birth, through gentle facilitation of woman-centred care.

In the leadership chapter, reference is made to a study (Byrom & Downe 2010) that reveals midwives' views of 'good' midwives and 'good' leaders, where similar descriptions were given of the two phenomena, especially around emotional capability. There are also the findings of a review of the literature of transformational leadership where a link is made to the philosophies of woman-centred care. Leading and influencing by example is a key element of successful leadership, but some midwives may never witness a positive role model. For this reason, the chapter includes descriptive accounts of midwifery and maternity services leaders who have successfully influenced practice and enhanced care for mothers and babies. Finally, Mary Renfrew uses the subject of breastfeeding to highlight the fact that success depends on all members of the team, and she suggests that successful leadership includes having the confidence to ask others to follow, the ability to work in collaboration, and to follow others.

Expertise

When defining expert practice, the main schools of thought seem to fall into two camps. On the one hand, cognitive researchers working largely from an epistemological position of positivism have examined the effect of repeated practice, and of methods of organising and retrieving memory on expertise. On the other hand, phenomenologists working from an interpretivist stance have sought to describe the nature of expertise as it is manifest in actual practice. There seems to be general agreement that experts learn effectively from past experience, and that they have rapid access to that experience in some form, such as chunking or cognitive scripts. Experts also seem to have the capacity to fit historical patterns of experience into possible templates for current and future action in a more efficient way than non-experts. However, this does not explain the difference between those who are expert in one specific domain and those who seem to be able to transcend domains of practice.

The theory of adaptive expertise goes some way towards explaining the difference between technical experts, who may be novices in all areas but the one in which they are practised and efficient, and those who can translate their expertise between at least some domains. The components identified in the meta-synthesis of midwifery expertise described in Chapter 6 may be useful in describing elements of expertise that are likely to cross domains, and to be strongly expressed in adaptive experts in healthcare. These components of wisdom, skilled practice, enacted vocation and connected companionship are not confined to or even, necessarily, present in midwives or other professionals who are trained within formal systems of education. As Ann Davenport illustrates, there is much to be learned from traditional midwives, particularly in terms of their understanding of the cultural complexities of their local context.

Those seen as experts in maternity care seem to value connected relationships with women and colleagues. This relationship is founded on mutual respect, honesty and trust. It is facilitated through giving women time, listening and through effective communication and presencing. As both Denis Walsh and Ann Davenport illustrate in Chapters 7 and 8 respectively, education and training can facilitate expert practice. However, this needs to be more than just the imparting of facts. Attitudes, prior experiences and individual values and beliefs of the health professional may significantly influence practice, which in turn may affect birth outcomes and women's experiences of care. Through reflection and critical evaluation of practice, both of these authors propose innovative approaches to developing and recognising expertise.

Collaboration

As maternity care in well-resourced countries becomes increasingly diverse, with provision in a range of settings and by a range of practitioners, effective collaboration takes on increasing significance. Equally, in resource-poor settings where timely and efficient transfer is essential to deal with the epidemic of maternal mortality, collaborative working is fundamentally important. Women and babies who are transferred between settings are more likely to experience an adverse outcome than those who remain in one setting, particularly where different philosophies of care exist in the two locations (David *et al.* 2006). There are examples of initiatives where both maternal mortality and caesarean have been dramatically reduced (Soguel 2009). In these cases, the active element seems to be effective boundary work, in which the cultural, practice and philosophical differences between the local community base and the central referral hospital have been actively addressed.

This suggests that authentic collaboration is more than simple team-working. To build effective collaboration in maternity care, practitioners require willingness to cross sticky boundaries between disciplinary groups, whether professional or traditional, whether based on radically different philosophies of care, and even where there are contrasting beliefs about what is science and, therefore, what is evidence-based practice. As has been noted in Chapter 9, the development of communities of practice, based on positive (salutogenic) principles, may be one route to achieving this goal. Communities of practice cannot be artificially created. They grow from the engagement of people with a common interest and vision. Even if they don't agree on all the details of how to achieve the vision, those who coalesce into a community of practice will share mutual trust, belief in the end goal, and a willingness to innovate and to work together even in difficult and challenging circumstances. In other words, they exhibit genuine collaboration. The case studies across the whole book illustrate these characteristics perfectly, demonstrating that communities of practice exist informally in a range of circumstances. They, and the collaborative relationships they are built on, are the engines for positive change in maternity care, as they are in a wide range of other areas of health and social care.

Conclusion

The contributors to this book have offered a range of theoretical, philosophical and practical insights into leadership, expertise and collaboration. As editors, we firmly believe that optimal well-being for women, babies, families and the practitioners caring for those who use the maternity services is most likely to occur when transformational leadership, adaptive expertise and authentic collaboration are in evidence. We accept, however, that there are other ways of believing and practising in these areas. We hope the scholarship and debate in the book have challenged and intrigued you, the reader, and that you will continue reflecting on these important areas of your practice into the future.

References

Byrom S, Downe S (2010) 'She sort of shines': midwives' accounts of 'good' midwifery and 'good' leadership. *Midwifery* 26(1): 126–37.

David M, Berg G, Werth I, Pachaly J, Mansfeld A, Kentenich H (2006) Intrapartum transfer from a birth centre to a hospital – reasons, procedures, and consequences. *Acta Obstetrica et Gynecologica Scandinavica* 85(4): 422–8.

International Congress of Midwives (2010) *Young Midwifery Leaders Programme.* www.internationalmidwives.org/Projects/YoungMidwiferyLeadership Programme/tabid/334/Default.aspx (accessed June, 2010).

Osbourne A (2004) A culture of fear: the midwifery perspective. *Midwifery Matters* 100, Spring.

Royal College of Midwives (2010) *Midwifery Leadership Programmes.* www.rcm.org. uk/college/professional-development/midwifery-leadership-programmes/ (accessed June, 2010).

Soguel D (2009) Gravity birth pulls women to Ecuador hospital. *WeNews,* February 15th 2009. www.womensenews.org/story/health/090215/ gravity-birth-pulls-women-ecuador-hospital (accessed June, 2010).

Index

Essential Midwifery Practice: Leadership, Expertise and Collaborative Working,
first edition. Edited by Soo Downe, Sheena Byrom and Louise Simpson
Published 2011 by Blackwell Publishing Ltd.
© 2011 Blackwell Publishing Ltd.

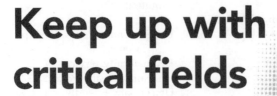
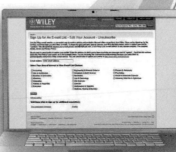